Praise for *Bloo*

"Sharing a raw, honest look at facing and enduring a history of trauma, *Bloodlines* shows that the road to recovery is paved with acceptance, hope, and love. Yokas's story, told with power and warmth, will help parents who are navigating mental health crises understand that the chains that bind us up in narratives often were forged long before we were born—and that they can be broken."

—BookLife Reviews, Editor's Pick

"*Bloodlines* will take you on a journey into the heart of a mother's love, but it's not a straight line. Circling through the generations, through patterns of being lost and found, Tracey manages the rough road of her daughter's adolescence and finds that the question *What is best for my child?* may not be the only one to ask. This is a brave story about how we find ourselves while we are looking to heal our children."

—Linda Joy Myers, founder of the National Association of Memoir Writers and author of *Don't Call Me Mother* and *Song of the Plains*

"We hear the harrowing statistics about kids with sky-high rates of anxiety and depression and the tendency to self-harm, and we immediately want to do something to help these children—but in our rush to empathize, we often forget the other part of mental illness: the mom's story. What is it like to love someone in so much pain, and to parent them through it? In this unflinching memoir, Tracey Yokas gives us that tale. It is a story filled with pain and with hope, told with generosity and love."

—Jennie Nash, founder and CEO of Author Accelerator

"This book will help parents who are navigating their child's mental health crisis know that they're not alone . . . but it also illuminates this fact: no matter what is breaking your heart, sometimes the best place to look for answers is inside yourself. Tracey Yokas shows us how."

—Laura Munson, *New York Times* and *USA Today* best-selling author of *This Is Not The Story You Think It Is* and *Willa's Grove*; founder of acclaimed Haven Writing Programs

"Tracey Yoka's masterfully and emotionally weaves the tale: a daughter's mental health diagnoses and a mother's quest to support her. *Bloodlines* is a raw, honest look at the limitations a history of trauma can have on us and our loved ones. A painful and arduous road to recovery—for both mom and daughter—is also a testament to acceptance, hope, and love."

—Jeni Driscoll, author of the mental health blog *Peace from Panic*

"In her journey to examine and understand the emotional scars handed down from her family experience, Tracey Yokas finds her truth and her voice. We witness the beautiful unfolding of powerful insight, courage, and wisdom. Tracey becomes a warrior to free her daughter, herself, and her family from a tangled web of illness and trauma."

—F.D. Raphael, author of *The Rock Stars of Neuroscience* and founder of MindfulnessbyFaithe.com

"In this painful but ultimately luminous memoir of motherhood and intergenerational healing, Tracey Yokas retraces—with unflinching clarity and steadfast devotion—her adolescent daughter's descent into disordered eating and self-harm. Ultimately, what Yokas discovers in her quest to help her daughter heal through unconditional love and compassion, is that she, too, is worthy of the same. A glorious, intricate, and astutely artistic exploration of the ways in which we live, love, overcome, and sometimes even triumph, not in spite of, but because of, our human fragility and imperfection."

—Jeannine Ouellette, author of *The Part That Burns*

BLOOD LINES

BLOOD LINES

A MEMOIR OF HARM AND HEALING

TRACEY YOKAS

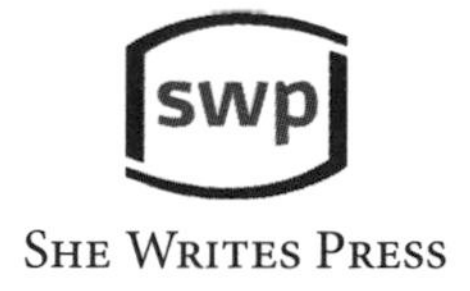

SHE WRITES PRESS

Published 2024

Printed in the United States of America
Print ISBN: 978-1-64742-345-2
E-ISBN: 978-1-64742-346-9
Library of Congress Control Number: 2021921421

For information, address:
She Writes Press
1569 Solano Ave #546
Berkeley, CA 94707

Interior design and typeset by Katherine Lloyd, The DESK

She Writes Press is a division of SparkPoint Studio, LLC.

Names and identifying characteristics have been changed to protect the privacy of certain individuals.

For my daughter

For the ones who feel alone

AUTHOR'S NOTE

The people, places, and events depicted here are as true to my memory as possible. In order to preserve anonymity, a few names, and in certain cases identifying details, have been changed.

A scar is concise communication.

—Maggie Smith

PREFACE

I stared at the cobalt-blue velvet bag on Mom's kitchen counter, imagining the sand-like ash mixed with leftover bone bits inside. I ached to rip it open, to sift through the grain, feel the calcified edges pressed into my palm. To what end? Knowing my mother, now dead, somehow better than before?

I was supposed to be in the car on the way to the airport and my flight home to my family in California. I'd been at Mom's place for the better part of a month dealing with the aftermath of her stroke and subsequent death: notifying, organizing, crying. I was ready to leave, but my legs refused to carry me out the front door. The velvet bag was a magnet.

Meanwhile, early morning sunlight filtered through a canopy of leafy trees in the backyard. I walked into the living room to take another look around. Shadows danced across the carpet. I loved the view beyond the glass. Mom had loved it too—all of nature's greens, especially at this time of year. Later, the cicadas would shrill their summer song and herald the end of another steamy hot New Jersey day. By then, I'd be long gone.

Heaviness settled in my chest. I sensed that I might never see this place again, that Mom's longtime boyfriend, Bob, with whom she'd been living for twenty years, would sell the condo and make a change after losing her. They'd been planning to move anyway, with Mom due to retire soon. They'd jaunted to Florida, one or the other of the Carolinas, and Austin searching for the perfect spot to nurture a final roost. *Damn it.* Mom was only sixty-seven years old when she died. She'd already survived two bouts of breast cancer and a double mastectomy. Just a month ago, we'd been chatting about her upcoming visit to see Faith's play—Mom adored her thirteen-year-old grandchild, her only one—and the very next day Bob had called from the car on the way to the hospital.

Life skidding off course. Again.

Dad had died six years earlier. Now, both my parents, gone. I felt adrift.

I didn't grow up in this house. Still, everywhere I looked brought good memories flooding in. Here, Faith had smushed her mouth and face with cake and ice cream when she turned one. There, Faith had cupped her ears against one of my favorite things: a deafening thunderstorm. Outside, Faith had chased her first firefly and scissored her first snow angel. Colorful Easter eggs, fat, fluffy Christmas trees, and gasp-worthy Fourth of July fireworks. And right beside us, laughing and engaged, Mom.

Mom had acted differently with Faith than she had when I was a kid. With each reunion, Faith had catapulted herself into my mom's open arms. They'd cuddled on the couch watching *Scooby-Doo* cartoons and playing board games, and had explored the great outdoors. Mom had rolled up her sleeves, gotten messy. Play-Doh. Paint. Science experiments. Flour. Snow balls in her house! I couldn't believe some of the things Mom tolerated, and even enjoyed, with Faith.

"I wouldn't have gotten away with that," I'd say.

"I've changed," Mom would say.

And now, I worried about what to expect at home. My husband had broken the news to Faith while I was en route. Theo, eighteen years my senior, was experienced with grief's many disguises, having already lost both parents and his first wife. He'd told me over the phone that Faith had said, "Okay," then walked away. She had always been a sensitive child, so her stoicism had unnerved us both. I'd wanted to protect her. I'd thought seeing the coffin and the body and enduring a full Catholic Mass combined with feeling pressured about how to act in front of strangers would be too much for my daughter. And knowing how much Mom had cared about looks, I felt certain she would have abhorred Faith's final vision of her being a stiff, lifeless shell. "Why upset the apple cart?" I'd said to Theo, and he'd agreed. But in retrospect, I couldn't shake the feeling that I'd stolen something from Faith, not least of which was the chance to say goodbye.

As I ruminated on a choice I could no longer change, I wandered into the TV room. Mom's travel and décor magazines, neatly stacked, awaited attention. An indentation like a cupped hand in the couch cushion where she always sat. Photos on the shelf. I grabbed one, wiped dust off the glass. Mom with three other relatives, arms draped across shoulders, evergreens and shiny wet pavement littered with lemon-yellow leaves. She dyed the gray out of her cropped brown hair, had zero wrinkles, quit smoking a long time ago, kept her weight down, and exercised regularly. Such vitality. But underneath her smile, underneath the carefully curated exterior, I detected our history, a legacy that had impacted her, our tiny family, and me those many years ago—my baby sister's stillborn death, my parents' grief and depression, their failed marriage. And about all of it: silence. Consequences had slithered into every nook and cranny of our lives. For decades, I'd been holding onto questions I'd meant to ask, but now there would be no answers.

I carried the photo to the kitchen. Bob was waiting for me in the car, and I didn't want to miss my flight. But that velvet bag of ash. I knew Bob would take good care of it—of her—until he drove out to California, where, at her request, we would commit her ashes to the sea. In the meantime, there was nothing left to do but get back to living.

I shoved the photograph into my purse and headed for the door.

The next evening, alone amidst a small crowd, I sat in the auditorium watching Faith's final performance in the musical *Aladdin Jr.* Theo had deferred, having already attended several of the previous shows. Around me, moms, dads, grandparents, siblings. Everyone smiling, happy. Onstage, an Arabian-themed cardboard set, exotic music, kids singing, more kids dancing. Red lighting implied a hot desert environment.

Faith, who would start eighth grade at summer's end, had already been acting for six years and usually hated playing a boy. But not this time. She crept out from behind the curtain, as Aladdin, the lead. Adorable, dressed in a brown vest, purple harem pants, and red fez and cummerbund. Thick brown hair, like mine and Mom's, was cut to her chin. Fake dirt streaked her face. She scampered across the stage with just the right amount of boyishness, joined the chorus in song. Buoyant energy, a mischievous grin. Maybe I'd made the right decision keeping her home after all. Earlier, when I'd asked if she wanted to talk about what had happened to Grandma, she'd shaken her head. I'd expected tears, anger, or both, but she'd seemed more or less fine, and I'd dropped the subject. Now, she sounded great, looked confident, and commanded the stage.

I tried to relax into the unfolding drama: a princess outside the palace compound, bucking rules and disobeying her father. The normalcy soothed my frayed nerves. But the heat in the place was real. August. Southern California. No air-conditioning. Sweat beaded above my upper lip. Distracted, I fanned myself with my program. The seat next to me, where Mom should have been sitting, gaped like a giant black hole. My thoughts floated away.

Nothing had gone the way it was supposed to. Mom had survived the stroke. She was supposed to live. I'd flown out there to be by her side. Diligent. Ready to do whatever needed to be done. For a week, sitting beside the motorized bed, first in the hospital and then the rehab facility, I'd held her hand, babbling about nothing in particular, *NCIS* episodes running nonstop on the television. She couldn't eat or drink or speak. A feeding tube snaked up her nose and down her throat into her stomach. She'd stared at me, her mouth set in a straight line. Cheeks slack. Bruises, in shades ranging from green to black, bloomed across her hands, up her arms. I'd never seen her like that, not even remotely. Recovery was going slowly, but it was going, and sometime during that week I'd quit my job as a human resources professional. The plan was I would visit as often as possible. Give Bob a break. Help out. But at that moment, next to her bed, there was Faith's play to consider. Theo's freelance gig. "I promise I'll be back soon," I'd explained, stroking her cotton-soft palm.

Guilt had crushed my chest like a boulder. Guilt for leaving Mom. *Shitty daughter.* Guilt for being away from my daughter. *Shitty mother.* Impossible. Mom's eyes had met mine. She'd wanted me to know something, but I had no idea what. That yearning, the vulnerability of it, had shaken me, and I'd stood to leave. "I love you," I'd said, kissing her droopy cheek.

I never saw my mother alive again.

In the auditorium, people around me clapped, so I clapped too. Faith bopped and ran, hopped and posed. From my seat, I could see the cute dimple in her cheek. She made a joke. *Good delivery.* Flashed a thumbs-up, and, yep, people laughed. *Phew.* I fanned myself faster. Someone, one of the dozens of involved medical professionals, should have foreseen Mom's heart attack. I should have gotten back in time, but she died while I was on my way. *I should never have left. Was she wondering where I was? Was she terrified?* Tears threatened. I clenched my jaw.

When Mom's childhood best friend appeared at the wake, she'd looked at me, in the only black dress I owned that fit, a tiered sheath under a cropped jacket, just a touch of bling at the shoulders. "That looks like something I'd wear to a nightclub," she'd said. I'd fled back to my seat by the coffin.

When the priest gave the Mass, he'd ridiculed the red dress I'd chosen for Mom to wear—something about his tone and a lady in red, waiting, at the pearly gates. But she looked beautiful in bright colors. And she was 100 percent Polish. Had he never seen a Polish flag?

When my aunt, married to Mom's only brother, called solely for the purpose of giving me shit for not adequately consulting my uncle about the arrangements.

Damn it. Why were my best efforts never good enough?

Onstage, a blue satin–clad genie was doffing his chapeau, and my thoughts circled back around to the wake, standing next to Mom's body. Her female coworkers had lined up to shake my hand, tell me about my mother. *Lauraine was a gem. She was the first person I called after my cancer diagnosis. Lauraine helped me so much; she really supported me.* I'd known nothing of how my mother had shared herself with folks who'd needed help. I'd nodded, smiled, said *thank you* and *yes*. That was Mom. So helpful. Genuine. And it seemed to me now, watching my daughter "fly" beside a kid playing a magic carpet, that Mom had always been this way: a different type of person out in the world than she was at home. Why had the woman who so readily and so easily let her guard down with them never been able to with me, her own daughter?

I shook my head. I just needed to get through the next few weeks. Unemployed, privileged that Theo's salary would keep us afloat, I would, until school started, concentrate on Faith. I'd support her through the loss of her grandmother, like I had when my dad had died. She was so much younger then. But we would talk, if she wanted. Or not. Take in a movie, a trip to the beach—Faith's favorite place. Maybe go to the Santa Barbara Zoo, like we'd planned to do with Mom. Before. Marvel at the animals, ride the train, feed the giraffes. Then, school. At thirteen, she no longer needed me the way she used to. Mom and Dad were dead. I'd grieve, whatever that meant exactly, and I would figure out a way forward.

Suddenly, the music was hitting crescendo, kids bowing. The audience whooped and hollered. I joined in, and, when Faith ran into the spotlight, I jumped up and cheered.

At home, several days later, I stood in front of the open refrigerator extracting sliced turkey, cheese, mustard: lunchtime for Faith and me. She was old enough to make her own lunch, and normally a mundane task such as this would have annoyed me, but after the events of the prior month, I reveled in the simplicity.

I piled the sandwich ingredients on the counter, grabbed the bread and two plates. Faith walked in, her hair tucked behind her ears. "Just half today, please," she said, her blue eyes radiating residual energy from the performances. "And an apple instead of cookies."

"Okay, babe," I said, surprised. "Good choice." In this household, fruit was no one's first preference, but I didn't give her request another thought.

"And I need more nail polish remover. We're out." She headed toward her room.

"Yes, ma'am." Faith and her girlfriends loved to paint their nails.

I delivered Faith's plate and then I made my meal: a full sandwich with a heaping side of sour cream & onion potato chips. For dessert, I planned to eat those cookies Faith had decided to bypass.

The stress of Mom's death was causing me to eat more than I should, again. My size 14 pants were getting snug. I cared. Also, I didn't care. My mother had died. I deserved to eat whatever I wanted.

I popped a chip in my mouth; my taste buds pinged their thanks. I'd been dieting for thirty years, had tried almost every available name-brand plan, and some, like Weight Watchers and Jenny Craig, many times over. But there was also Overeaters Anonymous, Nutrisystem, Lindora, and the drug fen-phen before they realized it might cause heart valve damage. And alternative options like over-the-counter diet pills and hypnosis. I'd considered liposuction, until someone I knew who'd done it explained the recovery process.

Since middle school, I'd lost and gained the same twenty to thirty pounds, what? Ten or more times? My goal weight remained perpetually beyond my grasp. History dictated that soon enough I'd get sick of my too-big body and start whipping my fat ass back into some semblance of shape. But not yet. For today, I munched on my lunch and allowed myself the opportunity to sit there, lost in thought.

Two framed paintings of calla lilies, my wedding flower, hung on the dining room wall, reminding me of the engraved serving set Theo and I had used sixteen years prior to cut our wedding cake. Ceramic handles shaped like the lily. Gifted to us by Mom. *Oh, Mom.*

Tenacious and resilient, Mom could also be judgmental, shallow about appearances, and self-absorbed, and I hadn't lived up to her exacting standards. It was no mistake that my first major post-college adult decision had wrenched three thousand miles between us. I'd blamed her for whatever went wrong in our relationship—she was the adult, I the child. But after Faith had come along, I'd wanted her to know her only surviving grandparents—an opportunity denied me four times over. Carefully, watchfully, so as to protect my daughter from the negative messaging I'd received as a kid, particularly about my body, I'd regulated our time together and Faith had gotten Mom's best.

I shoved the last bite of sandwich into my mouth. A wave of disappointment washed over me. In my mother. In myself. I'd taken my parents' twenty-year age gap for granted, assuming that Mom, the younger of the two, would live at least as long as Dad had, to age eighty. Hubris. Why had we ignored the trouble between us, held our true selves back from one other? In effect, hid.

PART ONE

REGULAR ROUTINE

"I don't need breakfast," Faith said, surlier than usual. She was leaning against the kitchen counter, her arms crossed, her eyes bored. Her one-time request for less food two weeks earlier had become a regular routine: half sandwiches at lunch, no seconds at dinner, no snacks, and no desserts. I could already tell she'd lost weight.

Faith was by no means fat, but her pediatrician had been talking to me for almost a decade about her higher-than-average weight. At first, ashamed of my indulgent tendencies, I'd vowed to be stricter. I was an overweight kid; I didn't want that life for my daughter. Without explanation, I'd tried going at times to great lengths to divert, distract, alternately engage and deny. The silence was the opposite of what my parents, particularly Mom, had done by commenting about the food I ate, what I should have been eating instead, and generally what should be done about the problem of my body, which in my young mind equated to the problem of me. It was a pattern I'd refused to repeat.

But at other times, like when my little girl said she was hungry, what was I supposed to do? I didn't want to deny either one of us.

Cool morning air wafted in the open kitchen window behind me. "I'm glad you're getting your eating on track," I said, "but you still have to eat. Breakfast is important!"

"I'm not hungry."

I changed tack. "You're going through puberty, exercising a lot." Four days a week, Faith swam laps for an hour for summer swim team. We locked eyes. "You need adequate calories."

"I know," she said, walking away.

And so we went about our remaining summer plans. On August 14, I celebrated my forty-fourth birthday—my first birthday without my parents. I must have had thoughts and feelings about moving forward through life without them, and Theo probably whipped up a delicious dinner for the three of us. His culinary skills had always outshined mine. But instead, what I remember from those waning summer days was finding more of the meager amount of food that had been on Faith's plate in the trash.

Late one night, after Theo got home from work, I talked to him about Faith's new eating habits. "Don't worry, honey. She'll be fine, same as I was," he said, removing his heavy steel-toe shoes. "Remember, I told you I was teased, called ten-ton Tokas? Look at me now." It was true, he was fit and trim and healthy. Sober, having six years prior completed a twelve-step program. A former high school football player turned avid golfer, Theo doggedly maintained his athleticism, and his tone implied I was overreacting.

I *was* confused. Maybe my judgment was off. My experience with cutting back, on diets, was always strictly controlled as I ticked off boxes in a food diary, ounces of this and servings of that. Enough to eat, at least, always assured.

And I was a teenager and now an adult with friends who'd struggled with eating issues. I was a female in America, keenly aware of our destructive societal norms around weight, body image, dieting. Finally, I'd had some training. Spurred on by the kind words of a therapist, perpetually intrigued by what made people tick, still wondering why no doctor had thought to screen me for the postpartum depression that had hit me like a freight train after Faith's birth, I'd gone to grad school to get a master's degree in counseling psychology.

I had, in other words, questions. I scheduled a pediatrician appointment for before the start of school, just in case.

1977

Nowadays, there was so much good stuff on TV: *The Six Million Dollar Man*; *The Bionic Woman*; *The Love Boat*; *Laverne & Shirley*; *Three's Company*; *Charlie's Angels*; *M*A*S*H*; *All in the Family*; *The Incredible Hulk*; *Welcome Back, Kotter*; *CHiPs*; *Fantasy Island*; *Quincy, M.E.*; *Columbo*; and *The Hardy Boys*. Parker Stevenson and Shaun Cassidy were so cute! I said, "Ayyyy" like the Fonz, and braved long prairie walks alongside Laura Ingalls. Everything a nine-year-old could imagine! And more!

Sometimes Mom and Dad would watch with me. They sat next to each other on the couch, either holding hands or Mom draping her arm across Dad's shoulders. Dad, always on the lookout for his next joke, appreciated the funny shows with characters like that cranky Archie Bunker. Mom preferred stuff with some romance. At bedtime, one of them would say, "Up you go," and I'd head upstairs.

I loved to lie under my canopy, close my eyes, and see myself in the stories: leaping over fences with Jaime Sommers or solving mysteries with Frank and Joe Hardy. That was way more fun than worrying about Mom and Dad or feeling bad. I didn't know what I felt bad about exactly, why my stomach hurt so often for no apparent reason, why I threw up sometimes. Also for no apparent reason. But at nighttime, if I concentrated hard enough, as I drifted off to sleep, my fears melted into dreamy fantasies. I never did that with the big family shows, though, like *The Waltons* and *Eight Is Enough*. They made me jealous.

One or another of those Bradfords was always getting into trouble, just like one or another of the Waltons, but everything turned out okay by the end. They fought and they always made up. I assumed my life would be fun like that, interesting like that, if only I had a sibling. All my friends had siblings. I was my parents' only—the only only.

One day, Mom and Dad were in the kitchen. I was sitting on the couch with no one but my cat, Bumpy, for company. Sick and tired of being by myself, lonely, I wanted to be like everyone else. I wanted what they had. I marched up to my parents.

"I want a brother or a sister," I said. "Why don't I have one?"

Mom's face went slack. She sighed. She looked at Dad but didn't say anything. I waited for her to answer, but instead she walked away. She was always walking away, going to her room, being in one of her moods, staring out the window. It was like I was invisible. "What's wrong with her?" I asked.

"Your mother is not to be referred to as 'her,'" Dad said.

"Sorry," I said. I knew by now to be a good girl.

Dad pointed to a chair. "Sit down."

He explained that I had had a sister. "Her name was Lauren Patrice. She was born when you were two years old."

I didn't remember that. Not a single memory. I didn't remember Mom having a big stomach. I didn't remember tiny clothes or anyone talking about a baby. "What happened to her?" I demanded. "Where is she?"

"She died in the hospital before we could even bring her home. It was very, very sad, but there was nothing we could do. This is something we don't talk about. We mustn't upset Mom. Put it out of your mind and never bring it up again."

I sat there for a minute. I had so many questions, was trying to figure them out, but Dad told me to go watch TV.

"Okay, Dad," I said, sliding off the chair.

I headed for the couch, confused. I always did what Dad told me to, but why couldn't we talk about it? I was supposed to have a sister! I sat next to Bumpy. Stared at the big, empty, sooty fireplace. Dad had painted the rocks around the opening shiny white, but the area on top was stained black from smoke. Bookcases, packed with Dad's books, lined both sides. *I should have a sister.*

What would my sister look like? Would she like the same things I did? Would she want to watch shows with me? Draw with me? Having a little sister would make me a big sister. A big sister! I'd have someone to play with. Someone to watch out for. Someone to ride the bus with. To be mine. And I'd be hers. Instead, I had Bumpy.

I didn't understand how being quiet helped Mom because she was already upset. She was always upset about something. I could tell just by looking at her. Her face kinda scrunched up. She sighed. She smoked. She stared. She talked about making sacrifices for the family. *I must be selfish for wanting what I can't have.*

I remembered the fight Mom and Dad had had. They probably thought I couldn't hear because they'd closed the bedroom door. Why did parents not understand that kids could always hear, at least some of what they said, through a closed door? A door is just a piece of wood! Anyway, I was in my room, right across the small landing, sitting on the floor. I couldn't hear everything, but I'd heard enough.

"The whole point . . . family!" Dad had yelled.

". . . want us . . . just the two of us!" Mom had yelled.

The door had banged open. I'd flinched.

"Fine," Dad had said, storming downstairs, out the front door.

I'd stayed in my room, scared, hiding by my record player. I never told anyone what I'd heard. Eavesdropping was a no-no. But whatever the fight was about, one thing was clear: Mom didn't want me, and ever since then I'd been trying extra hard to be good, hoping not to say or do anything to make my parents mad.

ENOUGH, AT LEAST

Dr. Kay strode into the examination room, grabbed the folder from the pocket on the door, and looked at me. Faith sat on the table, frowning the way only a thirteen-year-old could. Eighth grade couldn't start soon enough.

"What's up? It's not time for a regular checkup yet, right?" the doctor asked. Her manner was crisp, like her creased khaki pants.

"No, her birthday's not until December," I said, sitting up straighter. "I thought we should come by. A lot's been happening. My mom died last month."

"I'm so sorry," Dr. Kay said.

"Oh, thank you. It was unexpected, and it's been hard." I glanced at Faith. Her frown morphed into a scowl.

"Okay," the doctor said, waiting.

I explained the cutbacks, exercising, and apparent weight loss. I felt awkward speaking for Faith, but the doctor needed the facts. "She needs to eat enough, at least," I finally said. "I figure she's sad about her grandmother, but she won't say much. This is all a big change." Familiar heat rose in my cheeks.

"Let's take a look." The doctor flipped Faith's chart open, checked the vitals recorded by the nurse. "She's five foot five and weighs one hundred thirty-four pounds. I see that's a ten-pound loss since your last visit." Which actually meant ten pounds in just the weeks since drama had ended.

"I'm fat," Faith said, matter-of-factly.

My heart sank. At some point, Faith had understood enough about my repeated conversation with the doctor to draw her own conclusions. But she was wrong, and my instinct kicked in. "You're—"

"Not fat," Dr. Kay said, finishing my sentence. Her eyes softened, and she rested a hand on Faith's knee. "You're so healthy, Faith. Doing great in every way." She continued to talk, and my thoughts drifted.

Five foot five, one hundred thirty-four pounds. I remembered a formula I learned somewhere, probably Weight Watchers, that said a five-foot-tall woman should weigh one hundred pounds, and you can add five pounds for each additional inch. I did the math. Theoretically, Faith's ideal weight was one hundred twenty-five pounds. Only nine pounds off the mark—a feat I couldn't relate to. She was definitely not fat.

I refocused on the doctor. "With the exercising, I want you to pay attention to eating enough protein. Add a handful of nuts into your daily routine. Keep a log if you forget what you eat. You can lose a couple more pounds, but you have to do it *very* slowly. Like, one pound over the next year."

Faith picked at the paper covering the exam table. "Kids are mean to me. They call me fat. I don't want to be fat anymore."

Back in sixth grade, Faith had admitted to being bullied. I'd demanded details, thought about barging into that elementary school and dressing down the principal—"What kind of joint are you running here, lady?"—but figured it wouldn't change anything. *Kids will be kids.* How often had I heard that? And when Faith had clammed up, I'd dropped it. I made a mental note to ask her more about the bullying now.

"Those other kids have the problem, Faith, not you," Dr. Kay said. "There's nothing wrong with you. You're a beautiful girl."

I nodded. But Faith looked skeptical. I wondered if there was a kid alive anywhere who'd avoided the scourge of bullying. I sure hadn't. *Thunder Thighs Tracey.*

The doctor patted Faith's knee. She appeared unconcerned. "Slow the weight loss waaaaayyyyyy down. Okay? And talk to your mom about how you're feeling. It'll help."

"Okay," Faith sighed.

From the doctor's office, we headed straight for Target and back-to-school shopping, merging onto the 101 Freeway. Our town, located forty miles north of downtown Los Angeles, sits nestled between the Santa Monica Mountain range's Boney Peak and Rancho Sierra Vista Park with its seven thousand acres of open land stretching for miles toward the ocean. "God's country," Theo always called it. Off to my left, old Boney and the hills, like outstretched arms, form a protective barrier that surrounded us in nature's beauty. I checked the doctor visit off my mental to-do list. *Get child to understand she needs to eat (without shaming, harping, or belaboring).* That was good parenting!

"Babe, about the bullying," I ventured.

"I don't want to talk about it."

"Okay, but the doctor's right, you know. You're perfect the way you are." She ignored me.

Outside, midday heat radiated off the asphalt. We exited the freeway, passed the Islands restaurant where we'd created a summer Monday night tradition. After Faith's active day at drama camp, we'd pop in for dinner, enjoying the Hawaiian vibe and delicious chicken sandwiches. I stole a sideways glance at her, my mom brain ticking off a quick list of positive traits: talented, kind, smart, funny, athletic, attractive. She wasn't seeing herself clearly. But what teenager did?

In Target, in the fitting room, Faith kicked off her sneakers, slid into a pair of junior size 13 jeans. They sagged like a poufy sack.

She smiled. "Can I try the next ones?"

I handed them over. Same result.

"I'll go get the next size down," I said.

I walked to the stacks with a bounce in my step. Faith was doing what I never could. In a couple of days, she'd start school wearing a cute T-shirt and smaller pants. There was nothing to worry about. She'd listen to the doctor's instructions, and her high school experience would be different than mine.

If this was the silver lining around the dark cloud of Mom's death, I'd take it.

MINING FOR DETAILS

I sat on the floor in front of my dresser, home alone. Faith was at school, Theo at work. Before I'd flown home from New Jersey, Bob had encouraged me to pack Mom's jewelry and anything else I'd wanted that would fit in my suitcase, and I'd stashed everything in the most convenient spot. Now, forlorn and lonely, with an urge to touch Mom's treasures, I opened the bottom drawer.

Calvin Klein jean jacket. I detected a hint of musky Opium perfume, ran my eyes over the blue denim, silver buttons, and size label, XL. But I'd never wear it; Klein's version of extra large was not nearly XL enough for me. A small heart-shaped pillow embroidered with flowers and the word *Mother*. I vaguely remembered giving it to her for a long-ago Mother's Day. There was a colorful "purse" younger Faith had made out of fabric loops on a kiddie weaving loom. Various boxes, plastic bins, and a small plastic tub that held most of her jewelry collection lined the bottom of the drawer.

My hand gravitated to one of the boxes. Inside, several vintage-looking brooches. I couldn't be sure, but I guessed they'd come to her from her mother, who had died when I was six months old. I was about to close the box when a tiny object, underneath the others, caught my eye. I gently poured the contents onto the floor. A small caduceus lapel pin—two snakes winding around a winged staff, traditional insignia of the medical profession.

Oh yeah. Mom had gone to nursing school. That would have been what? Like forty-five years prior to this. I rolled the pin between my fingers, digging down my memory pathways. She'd quit because a patient she'd grown fond of, a young man, had died. I knew at least that much of the story. Questions flooded my brain. I wanted to know who had given her the pin, if she'd ever worn it, and about her nursing aspirations, beyond the obvious. If there was more to the story of the young man who'd died? And Mom's father had apparently had a painful death, from what illness I did not know, when she was a girl of only seven or eight. Had his death factored into her decisions? Was her mother upset about her quitting?

The only word I could remember Mom using in reference to her mother was "tough." As in, "She was tough on us." The *us* being Mom and her younger brother, my uncle. When I was growing up, on the extremely rare occasions Mom had mentioned her childhood, in Brooklyn with a "tough" mother, I'd never mined for more details. But sitting on the floor now, holding the pin, I wondered about the expectations my grandmother may have had for my mother. About Mom's nature and nurture. What had made her the woman she became? And I imagined, yes, that in order to survive in New York in the 1950s, a single mother with two young children must have needed to be tough.

I scooped the brooches into the box, dropped the pin inside, and put the top on. I stored the box back in the drawer, replaced the "purse" and the pillow. I refolded the jacket. As I closed the drawer, I imagined Mom—nineteen or twenty years old—tucking out of sight and also nearby, forever, a reminder of what would never be.

THE HARD PART

Theo came home, threw his keys on the kitchen counter. It was two weeks into the school year. "We have a problem," he said, worry creasing his forehead. He'd just returned from repping us at back-to-school night, and I imagined, as I flicked dish soap from my fingers, that one of Faith's teachers had complained about her increasingly irritable attitude.

"Grace said that Faith's been throwing her lunches away," Theo said.

Grace was the mother of Faith's best friend, Isabelle. Isabelle was worried enough about Faith to break kid code and rat her out. Not good.

"Just this morning, Faith said she's eating her lunches," I said. "I asked her point-blank." But even as I spoke, I thought back to the way she'd screamed, "*Yes!*" and slammed her bedroom door in my face, the way I'd had to beg her to eat the broiled chicken breast and steamed broccoli dinner I'd made at her request. No breakfast, no lunch, and only a few bites of dinner—not enough.

Theo chucked his baseball cap onto the table. "I guess it's not true," he said.

Lying? I couldn't rule it out.

In sixth grade, Faith had swiped Theo's cell phone without

asking so she could fit in at school. Around the same time, we'd found out that she was showing up at her after-school program only to ditch and hang out with friends. Both times we'd questioned her, and both times she'd denied the allegations. Only when pressed had she confessed the truth. Theo had yelled at her about honesty, integrity, truthfulness, and reliability. So loud, in fact, that I'd intervened. Crying, she'd apologized. I'd chalked those incidents up to normal growing pains. But this was different.

"She has to eat," Theo said.

"I'll talk to her. Very soon. We have to nip this in the bud."

The next morning, I made Faith's lunch anyway. Shoved half a dry turkey sandwich and half an apple into a paper bag, folded it closed. When I peeked in Faith's room, she wasn't there. I looked across the hall into my room. She was in front of my full-length mirror, pulling and picking at her smaller clothes.

"You're disgusting," she growled at her reflection.

That was a first—I'd never heard Faith chastise herself this way.

"Babe," I said.

She whipped around. "You scared me."

"Sorry, I just—" I didn't know what to say. "Faith. You are *not* disgusting."

She blew by me into her own room, me trailing with the lunch bag.

"Just leave it," she said, jamming books into her backpack.

I placed the bag on her desk. "Babe, look at me, please."

"What? I have to finish getting ready."

"The car won't drive without fuel in the tank," I said. "Neither will your brain."

"I know. God. Can you leave me alone?"

"Can you watch the attitude?"

I understood how it felt to be thirteen and look in the mirror.

But geez. Faith had lost weight. The hard part was over. Except for how hungry she must have been, her attitude made no sense. I wanted to shake her or wrap her in my arms and smother her with kisses, the way I used to. When she was younger, she was always the first kid to strike a silly pose, make a funny face, act goofy. Her sense of humor was easy to delight in, but it dawned on me that I couldn't remember the last time I'd seen her smile.

I stepped into the hall. "We're not done talking about this. You can't sustain what you're doing. Human beings have to eat. Eat your lunch today."

She slammed the door in front of me. Again.

Another morning, preparing yet another lunch I hoped wasn't destined for the trash can, I heard Faith pad across the hardwood floor between her room and ours. *Now what?*

I tiptoed toward my room, my heart pounding. She wasn't there. I moved quietly toward the bathroom, then even more quietly into it. There she stood, on my digital scale.

"Fuck!" she shouted, jumping off. "You scared me."

My offense at her f-bomb didn't distract me from the readout: 127. I dug into my memory bank and pulled up the number from our trip to Dr. Kay's: 134.

The edges of the room went loose. *Is this . . . ?* A label—clinical, shockingly common for teenage girls—threatened to emerge into my consciousness. But I was afraid to acknowledge that thought, what a diagnosis might entail, and shoved it down deep. She just needed to eat, simple as that.

"You've lost more weight," I said. "Don't you remember what the doctor said? You have to slow it down."

She tried to walk by me, but I grabbed her arm. I wanted to drop a few f-bombs myself. I wanted to tell her to quit the fucking crap and to eat her fucking breakfast so we could move on with our lives. Two measly months had passed since Mom's death. I was depleted, had no patience. Faith's choice—because that's how it felt in the moment, like a choice not to eat—was driving me mad.

"What number's going to be low enough, Faith?"

She wrenched her arm free and left me standing there beside the scale.

1980

My doctor, Dr. Emma, was also a neighbor, which was kind of weird but also neat when I saw her in her driveway or at the store. My twelfth birthday wasn't until summer so it was too early for a regular checkup, and I hadn't thrown up in a while. I didn't know why we were there.

We stopped at the scale, and Dr. Emma asked me to step on. *Clunk*. She slid the metal thing to the right, to the right some more, and made a note in the folder she was holding. "Follow me," she said, heading toward her office.

Mom and I sat on our side of the desk. What a mess! There were loose papers and stacks of folders and junk all over the place. Mom would go nuts if my room looked like that.

Dr. Emma chitchatted with Mom for a minute, then turned her attention to me. "You need to lose thirty-five pounds," she said. I wondered if that was a lot. "You're in middle school, right? Sixth grade?" I nodded. "You don't want this problem getting worse."

Problem? I was a problem?

I looked at Mom. She was wearing her serious face. How could the problem get worse? I wanted to ask but didn't because it seemed like I should already know what Dr. Emma meant.

Dr. Emma handed Mom some papers. Mom and I listened as she said a bunch of stuff about eating less and skipping desserts and snacks until the weight came off.

"Basically, come up with something workable and stick with it every day until I say otherwise."

The same things? Every day?

"And get outside as often as possible. She spends a lot of time outside, right? Not watching television."

Mom's serious face rearranged into her frustrated face. She talked to Dr. Emma about the foods she cooked, how she tried. The word "but" hung in the air. She was disappointed in me, I could tell. And she said something about Dad buying me a sugary treat whenever I wanted one. I smiled because it was true. He did.

"We don't want the weight to follow her into high school," Dr. Emma said.

"I don't want the weight to follow her anywhere," Mom said.

Would I ever have ice cream or crumb cake again? Would Dad take me to Dairy Queen? Would Mom force me to eat that disgusting Veg-All she poured out of a can? I longed to be home with Bumpy, watching *B.J. and the Bear*, *Buck Rogers in the 25th Century*, or *Battlestar Galactica*. I did not like the idea of eating the same thing every day. Dad always said variety was the spice of life.

At home, I rushed upstairs to my room. Purple was my favorite color, and Mom had wallpapered in a lavender flower print. I grabbed my diary, flipped to a blank page, and shared the news. *I'm on a diet!* I wrote, like I'd won a contest.

Every night in my diary, I kept track of the shows I watched and what was happening on them. And I protected my secrets, like which boys I liked at school, and which girls I hated. I only hated a girl if a boy I thought was cute showed her attention. Every time a boy asked a girl out, I wrote it down. I told my diary which girls said yes or no. I tracked fights and breakups. All the boys were fighting over a girl named Karla. I was jealous, but I couldn't blame them. She was perfect, blond like Jaime

Sommers and Farrah Fawcett from *Charlie's Angels*. I looked nothing like them.

Soon I abandoned thinking about the diet, poring instead through the pages I'd written about other kids' busy social lives.

BIOLOGICAL IMPERATIVES

I moved through those early days, two months after Mom had died and after Faith went back to school, on autopilot. I walked from one end of the house to the other, passing pictures of us that were hanging on the wall, or sitting on the fireplace mantle, or out in the garage covering the tops of Theo's big, portable tool-filled work boxes. Loading clothes into the washing machine, over my shoulder, I could track our family timeline. Pre-marriage, Theo and me smiling on the red carpet in front of a life-size Oscar statue. Faith, barely three years old, atop the spring-mounted plastic horse Mom had bought for her one Christmas (Faith had ridden that thing so hard I feared the springs would snap, "Just like you did," Mom had said). Theo, in the bowels of the Kodak Theatre, when he was still the head carpenter there, pointing at the concrete wall where, to a height of twenty feet or so, he'd affixed at least a hundred, maybe more, of young Faith's drawings. Performers from around the world had had the opportunity to admire her squiggles, lines, suns, cats, and smiley faces.

Every time I saw *our* smiling faces, I felt utterly confused about why Faith wouldn't eat. How she could be fine one day and not fine the next day. At another time in my life, the answers may have been obvious. But, awash in grief and dismay, I couldn't make sense of it.

In my bedroom, straightening the comforter, in my mind's

eye, we were with Mom and Bob at Sundance riding the tram to the top of the mountain to pick wildflowers. Loading the dishwasher, we were at my Dad's, toddler Faith climbing into his lap for more cuddles. So ordinary. Or I'd find myself waking up, as if from a dream, in the grocery store in front of the pasta section or in CVS in front of the toothpaste. Worry combined with distracted rote motion reminded me of what life had been like when Faith was a baby. New, mewling, and needy. Perfect.

I'd thought I was prepared to be a mother. I'd read books about pregnancy, and Theo and I had taken classes about infant safety. As if. One day, I was a working woman, pregnant stomach out to there, but still. A real go-getter, the sort who, knowing no one, moves three thousand miles away from home to pursue a dream to work in the entertainment business and tenaciously starts achieving that dream. Seemingly the next day, they put a baby in my arms. What had I known about being a mother? About the ecstasy and the languor? The crippling insecurity? Or the love? Love such as I'd never imagined possible. My whole body had ached with it.

Postpartum depression had overtaken me almost immediately, although I hadn't understood for close to a year what was happening—lack of insight a common feature of mental illness. I'd cried whenever Faith had cried, and I'd cried on my own: in the shower, over the kitchen sink, in the backyard. I'd slept whenever she'd slept, which was hardly at all. I'd worried over every detail. Was my breast milk adequate? Should I supplement with formula? Should I change laundry detergent? Was that a cough? Could she tell how much I loved her? How dedicated was I? Was I doing enough?

I'd refused to let almost anyone besides Theo hold her. And when he'd returned to work and Faith and I were by ourselves and I'd had to take over bath time, meal making, and clothes washing, it had felt impossible to manage on my own. But I had buckled down, because that was what I knew how to do. Each day's sole purpose of caring for my daughter had carried me through to each night.

Now, as I put groceries away or headed for after-school pickup, I told myself, once again, to buckle down. For all my fear and anxiety back when Faith was a baby, she'd turned out fine. Better than fine. We'd been fine then, and we were sure to be fine again soon.

But a banana did us in.

It happened a few days after I caught Faith weighing herself on my scale, when she was getting ready for her evening hip-hop class. "You need to eat something before we leave," I said.

We were in my home office, next to the living room. "I'm not hungry, and I'm not gonna eat anything," she said, her fists planted on her hips. "I'm fat, Mom. Look at me."

I did look at her. Her shorts were almost roomy enough for a second person. The new school clothes I'd bought were already loose, and she'd eaten nothing all day. I steeled myself for a debate; Faith was used to hearing yes, getting her way. *Argue enough and Mom caves*—that was the typical pattern. Theo had often warned me, "Kids need to hear no once in a while." I knew he was right, but I couldn't help myself. I hated to disappoint my daughter.

Now, she had to be hungry. "I told you," I said. "No food, no class. You can't survive without food."

She stomped toward the kitchen. "I'm fine. You're making a big deal about nothing." The refrigerator opened, then the cabinet. "The other girls at school never eat anything."

"That's their mothers' problem."

My stomach churned at the thought of the girls I saw floating around the middle school campus—grape-shaped heads atop toothpick-thin bodies. Was anyone else concerned?

Faith returned with a banana and a glass of milk. I watched as she gobbled up the fruit, gulped down the liquid. She slammed the glass down on the coffee table. "Satisfied?"

"Yes, actually."

"I hope you're happy now," she growled. "I hate myself."

"Oh, brother. Let's go."

I grabbed my purse, feeling like I'd forced an entire cheesecake down her throat. By the time we got in the car, her words had penetrated my frustration. Did Faith really hate herself? Over a banana?

Twilight. The dance school parking lot was on a hill. I stared out the windshield, lights twinkling in the distance, arguing heatedly with myself. *This is serious. No, it's a phase. No. Problem.* How long could her brain properly function, I wondered, on so little food, so much exercise?

It was a beautiful evening, the sky transitioning to shades of orange, pink, and navy blue. Seeing the sunset reminded me of Hawaii. Faith's favorite place to visit, trips made possible by Theo's exceedingly long work hours. The two of them—Theo and Faith—with their Mediterranean skin. While I huddled nearby under a wide-brimmed hat, umbrella, towel, and SPF 70 sunscreen, they'd slather themselves with low SPF to crisp up in the sun. No matter her age, when Faith would say to Theo, "Let's go in," he complied. They slid down waterslides and bodysurfed and porpoised through the waves like the slick, shiny mammal. By day's end, their cheeks would be redder, the rest of their skin tanner, and we'd drag our chairs into position for the unfolding spectacle. Theo and I had both had childhoods shaped by financial insecurity, so we never took these trips for granted. Punch-drunk on sunshine and salt water, Faith would lay her head on my shoulder, drape her arm around me, and together, as the giant orb sank toward the horizon, we'd ooh and aah.

Now, I needed a sounding board, another opinion about how

far off track Faith had fallen. Or not. I didn't trust myself. Nor did I trust Theo—a man who, before getting sober, had lost thirty pounds in three months that time he quit beer for a while—to understand the nuances of teenage girls and food. Dr. Kay had said I could call if I needed her. Maybe I needed her. I dug my cell phone out of my purse.

As soon as I stopped spilling it all out, the phone clutched to my ear, Dr. Kay *tsked*. "This isn't good," she said. "She might be anorexic."

I burst into tears, the parking lot blurring all around me. The training I'd received in grad school had not prepared me, at all, for the reality of hearing these words spoken about my own daughter. I'd expected Dr. Kay to say *don't worry* or *she'll be fine* or *we'll get a handle on this*. My daughter could not have a mental illness. She could not be anorexic. Anorexics were walking skeletons; Karen Carpenter—waxen, fragile, and deranged from starvation. They were not my athletically inclined, poetry-writing, honor-class-taking, formerly food-enjoying daughter. I dug in my purse for tissues, came up empty.

"I want to get a few resources for you, but she may need to go into inpatient treatment," the doctor said.

I recoiled. "Inpatient treatment? This doesn't make sense." First Mom, now this. I blew my nose on my sleeve. "She was fine and now she's not. It's like someone flipped a switch. She just needs to eat."

"Bring her in again, and take care of yourself. I can tell this is really upsetting you."

We ended the call. I wiped my face with my sleeve, dug my makeup compact out of my purse, and swiveled the rearview mirror. I blotted my red nose and cheeks. Inpatient treatment was an outrageous first step. Ridiculous. But I'd never say that out loud—questioning authority figures was rude. I'd hear whatever the doctor had to say; after all, she had my daughter's best interests at heart. But I knew that more moderate options existed. I dabbed more powder across the bridge of my nose, covering up the evidence.

At the doctor's office, again. No idle banter, just confirmation that Faith had lost an additional seven pounds in the three weeks since the doctor had told her to eat more.

"I'm worried, Faith," Dr. Kay said. "Your stomach is almost concave."

"I told you—I don't want to be fat anymore," Faith said, her lips compressed into a thin line. "Look at this." She was wearing a bathing suit—up next, swim practice—and pinched a tiny bit of flesh covering her abdomen.

"You have to have skin, Faith!" Dr. Kay exclaimed. "What do you think keeps everything in place?"

I shook my head. I could pinch the flesh around my stomach and really show Faith something to be upset about. Her wristbones protruded like golf balls, and after swim she'd complain about feeling fatigued and in the next breath, the newest bit, that the workout wasn't hard enough. "I estimate she's getting maybe five, six hundred calories a day," I said. "Max."

"You've got body dysmorphia," Dr. Kay said. "You're misjudging your appearance. When was your last cycle?"

Faith had gotten her period two years ago, when she was in sixth grade.

"I don't know. Not this month," Faith said.

"Or last month," I said.

I'd heard of this condition: amenorrhea. Faith's food intake had already dropped low enough so that her body was unwilling to expend the energy to bleed. Her weight might not have dropped enough to require life-saving action, but things were adding up:

her habits were taking a toll on her emotional well-being, she wasn't seeing herself realistically, and she'd lost her period.

"I think it's time for you to get some help, Faith," Dr. K said.

Faith sat on the exam table like a stone, staring at the floor.

After Faith made a beeline for the pool deck, I sat in the shade on the sideline. On an ordinary day, I would have pulled out my book and settled in, enjoying the soft breeze and rumble of churning water. Almost like vacation. But this was no ordinary day. It was official: my daughter had an eating disorder.

I watched Faith cheerfully mingle with the other kids, seemingly oblivious to the conversation we'd just had with her doctor. Outside of school, she'd stopped hanging out with friends, no one came over anymore, and she turned down social activities in preference to doing calisthenics alone in her room. So, while Theo and I had considered pulling her off the swim team unless she agreed to eat more, that seemed harsher than was necessary. Water, whether ocean, pool, or shower, was Faith's happy place. And we were hoping the camaraderie of the swim team would help.

Faith stuffed her hair under a tight silicone cap, snapped a pair of goggles in place. In the moment, I couldn't help but compare her new slimmer outline to the other kids'. She had nothing to feel self-conscious about.

Coach blew the whistle. A couple dozen bodies jumped in the pool, started warming up with freestyle laps. At Faith's turn, she dunked under the water, kicked off the wall, and propelled forward like a spear. She broke the surface—reach, reach, reach and breathe and reach, reach, reach and breathe—settling into an easy rhythm. I marveled at her stamina. Effortlessly, she reached the lane's end, flipped, and zoomed in the opposite direction.

I'd swum, too, as a kid, and I could sprint like a Tasmanian devil. For twenty-five yards. Beyond that, forget it. I could never figure out how to go slow and easy, how to enjoy the feel of my body in the water, time my breathing. It was all or nothing. Usually nothing. The pressure of competition made me nauseous.

In the car with Dad, staring at the neighborhood lake, lane flags fluttering in the breeze, I'd often asked him to take me home. *I don't feel good.* He'd always complied. A crap lesson for a kid, in my adult opinion. I'd never let Faith quit, even back in kindergarten when, dutifully following the doctor's suggestion, I'd signed her up for the sports of her choice: soccer and softball. "Too hard, too hot, too sweaty, too dirty. I don't want to," she would sometimes complain. "Sorry," I'd say. "You don't have to join next year, but you have to follow through on your responsibility to the team." About this, Theo and I had agreed, and for five years, until Faith switched to swimming, she'd always signed back up.

In the tang of chlorine, kids clumped up at the far end of the pool, a swarm of wet bees, taking a breather, barely breathing heavily. While Coach talked, they hung from the wall, each other, lane dividers. Faith bobbed, her cap and goggles serving to highlight how much her nose and jawline resembled Theo's Greek heritage. Her body had to be screaming protestations: pangs, twinges, rumbles, gnawing, hollowness. She had to feel shaky, light-headed. That's what happened to me, anyway, whenever I'd drastically restrict my food intake and increase my activity level. How was she ignoring the biological imperative to eat?

Concerned as I was, residential treatment was a hard no, the idea downright offensive. Not only was it too soon, but also, years ago, a friend had told me about her own stint in an eating disorder facility. A twisted version of *who can eat the least and beat the system* kind of competition, she'd said. I imagined my daughter in a sterile setting like that, surrounded by devious skeletons, comparing see-through skin, brittle hair, jutting bones. No way. About this, Theo had also agreed.

Coach blew the whistle and off they went, again. Laps of butterfly: arms scooping, legs kicking, water flying. Faith barreled down the lane. I pulled out my cell phone, searched Amazon for *eating disorder.* Thousands of book titles to scan. Shame pulsed through me, my toes tingling. I'd tried so hard to avoid repeating my parents' mistakes specifically so that Faith wouldn't end up feeling about her body, herself, the way I felt about mine, myself. And back when I was in therapy, during Faith's early years, I'd talked to my therapist, who also happened to be my Weight Watchers leader, about my food habits, eating for emotional comfort rather than survival. And then there was grad school.

The program, three years of education and training, had focused on assessing people, circumstances, upbringing, and relationships. In other words: nurture. Our past. Familial history. The dynamics at play, the patterns and repetitive interactions that affect how we learn and who we become. In addition to genetics, our children's mental health and wellness, I'd learned, is strongly tied to the environment in which they are raised. My education, it seemed to me now, with a newly diagnosed child, had supported the gnawing sensation building in my gut: I was responsible. My best efforts, once again, had been nowhere near good enough. At the very least, I should have been able to see this coming and pivot.

Faith reached the lane's end, flipped, and rocketed forward. Butterfly is the most difficult stroke to master, but she effortlessly skimmed across the water. Impressive. Probably no one and nothing specific was to blame for my daughter's illness. Or, conversely, maybe everything was to blame: genetics, Theo and me, bullies, our looks-obsessed judgmental culture, social media. But when someone I loved hurt, I hurt. As a mother, I wanted to fix my daughter's pain. Fixing shit was *my* biological imperative.

1972

This place where Dad now lived was nothing like our nice, big house next to the lake. I was four years old and scared of New York City. It was smelly and noisy. Everyone honked their car horn. Bumpy had to stay home with Mom. I didn't understand why she was there and he had to live here. Nobody told me anything. The couch was different, ugly pictures were on the wall, and it was so small. I felt like I might cry, again. I cried all the time since Dad moved, but I scrunched my eyes. I didn't want to make him sad, so I tried to be brave.

"You stay here," Dad said, walking toward another room where I could see a bed.

He went into the bathroom, closed the door. I was too afraid to move. I heard the water turn on, then off. He came out wrapped in a towel, sat on the bed, all hunched over. His shoulders started to shake. Dad was crying. Dad never cried.

I went to him. "What's the matter, Daddy?"

"Oh, nothing." He changed his face around. "I'm sad for children who suffer."

Something in my stomach tumbled. He was sad, so I was too. I needed to help him, to take care of him the way he always took care of me.

I stroked his strong hand, fiddling with the gold ring he never, ever took off. No one else lived there. It was up to me.

"Don't cry," I said.

Smiling, he wiped his eyes. He kissed my cheek. He was always doing that. "You know what?" he said. "Let's have some ice cream. That'll make us feel better."

I clapped. Ice cream was my favorite.

In the kitchen, Dad got the carton from the freezer.

"Strawberry," I said.

"Right-o," he said.

He handed me the bowl and a spoon. The first bite stung my tongue, and soon we were laughing and laughing.

THE ONLY TYPE OF MEMORY I WISH WE HAD

"Come here, but be quiet," I beckoned to Faith.

We were in her bedroom. In this memory, she was six years old or eight or ten or twelve because every year the hummingbirds returned. I was next to the window that looked into the backyard, venetian blinds lowered and louvered closed, and she'd just caught me peeking like a nosy neighbor between the dusty slats.

Every spring a mama would construct her nest in the ficus tree directly outside the back door. The location made no sense; we used that door numerous times a day. But each year the drama unfolded in much the same way. First, in the living room, through the open window behind us, Faith and I would hear telltale chirps and hums. We'd see the sway of a thin, nubby branch or the blur of a bullet-fast body. But to actually see her, her wings spread phoenix-like, hovering in a state of suspended animation, required diligent patience. It required waiting, stock-still, staring through the glass at the exact spot among the branches where bits of twig, pieces of leaf, and tendrils of cat hair were accumulating.

Sometimes, when mama was foraging, I tiptoed outside. Unless you knew exactly where to look, the fruit of her labor was imperceptible—a home that, once complete, would amount in mass to the size of a quarter and in weight to a piece of paper. Faith would join me and we'd bend, twist, and crane to see, climbing, carefully, onto a chair to peer between the leaves, avoiding contact with any part of the tree. We were obsessed with tracking her progress.

Then, one day, the treasure would appear: two jelly-bean-size eggs.

Time to incubate.

Mama sat on the nest. We closed the windows, the curtains, the blinds. Turned down the television volume. Theo did his part too, avoiding the back door, taking the long way around to open the outside fridge or use the hose. We worked as a family to keep them safe, Faith fretting over errant noises, predators. "The mama might get scared or hurt! She might abandon the eggs! We have to protect them!" Stealthy squirrels. Screeching jays, whose jarring *caw-caws* propelled us outside to locate said interlopers and, at a distance from the ficus, chase them, and any invisible threats, away by jumping up and down, yelling, "Shoo!" and pinwheeling our arms. No act was too dorky or too brazen to protect our tiniest family members.

One year, in yet another attempt to scare away the jays, behemoths compared to our delicate hummingbirds whose iridescent green feathers practically glowed, Theo climbed up a ladder onto the roof, where the jays would alight, to screw in place a battery-operated, motion-sensor hawk. When triggered, it made a *keeeeee* sound and the eyes flashed red. The whole endeavor gave us a sense of control.

What joy when our babies made their way into the world! Elation! And I chose to believe the mamas knew we were on their side. That trust in us was why they always returned to nest in a less than ideal spot.

I had never considered myself a keen observer of nature until I became a mother and wanted to share the circle of life with my daughter. As the years passed, Faith's care and concern for our feathered family members grew, and she began on her own to watch, shelter, protect. She'd stand guard, clear away detritus, and corral the cats. Watching her dedication, I thought, *What a magnificently sweet person you are.* And, *How did I get so lucky to be your mom?* I had no trouble imagining her future: whatever Faith might choose to nurture would, with her vigilance and guidance, grow and flourish. And on the days in those years when fate intervened, when our best attempts failed, when an unseen disaster occurred and all that remained in the morning was an empty space where the nest and its vulnerable inhabitants had rested, we clung to one another and wept.

But that day in Faith's room, when I told her to come here, she took her place beside me. The tree was several feet beyond the window, and I handed her my camera, telephoto lens attached, slowly spreading apart the aluminum slats. I knew what she'd see, because I'd already seen it. Scraggly little baby heads lolling, mouths gaping, and mama, perched on the edge of the nest, gliding her long, thin beak into their heartbreakingly small beaks.

It took Faith a second to spot them. "Oh, Mama," she said. She meant me, not the bird.

"I know," I said.

We stayed that way, bound by awe, until mama hummingbird darted away to restock on nectar.

MEMORIES WE ALSO HAVE

Halloween

Halloween ranked up there with Christmas. Faith was six years old, in first grade, and she and her little bestie, Mia, were in Faith's room playing. I was in the kitchen with Mia's parents, Evelyn and Tony, putting the final touches on the dinner preparations—my special chili recipe, bubbling like witch's brew, had been simmering since dawn. Next to the range top, a ceramic bowl, a clawed gray hand exploding from the center, overflowed with mini-size Snickers, Kit Kats, and 3 Musketeers. Outside, Theo was filling the fog machine with special fog-making fluid. Laughter echoed down the hallway—the girls hopped up from the elementary school costume parade, lots of sugar, and the promise of more to come.

"Girls," I called out, "soup's on."

Feet thundered down the hallway. Theo came in, dropping a pair of work gloves on the counter. "Ready!" he said.

We filled our bowls, settled around the table.

Theo and Tony made small talk about work. Mia screeched, seeing a small black spider under her napkin. Fake. I'd covered the orange-and-black checkered tablecloth with them, spindly plastic legs on the butter dish, under forks, cradled in spoons. She took a bite of chili. "This is good," she said, long blond hair framing her face, freckles dotting her nose. She looked every bit the part she'd soon be playing as Alice in Wonderland.

"Yummy," Faith said.

I was tickled pink. I looked at Evelyn, who, it was clear, was also enjoying herself. Finally, I could let my guard down.

My decision, six years prior to this, to quit my career and stay home with infant Faith had been an agonizing one. I'd finally stepped a few rungs up the success ladder when: baby. And, along with her, the gift of a choice. I'd never once regretted prioritizing my daughter. But adjusting hadn't been easy.

For one, friendships. Women I'd hung out with before were either still working or lived too far away for mall meetups or shared Mommy & Me classes. Twice, over the last six years, I'd met women who seemed to want and need companionship as much as I did. Twice, I'd thought I made a solid friend. Twice, for reasons I still didn't fully understand, the friendships had fallen apart. Then I met Evelyn when she signed Mia up in kindergarten for my Girl Scout troop. I'd been reluctant at first, protective of my heart, but Evelyn's persistent niceness had worn me down. Now, here we were. A holiday, together. I leaned back, soaking in the tableau.

Six of us around our table breaking bread, happy. It was perfect, and the first of what I hoped would become an annual tradition.

"Mia's costume is fantastic," I said, relieved to remember the compliment.

"Thanks," Evelyn said. "I was at the sewing machine all last week finishing it."

Faith, meanwhile, would soon slip back into her store-bought red devil dress and plastic horn headband.

Theo, swigging his beer, asked Tony a question about his job as a fireman.

Tony swallowed. "Well—"

"What's that job like?" Faith interrupted.

"Faith," Theo snapped. "Don't interrupt."

Faith looked at her bowl, crestfallen.

"She's just curious," I intervened.

Tony shot Evelyn a look.

Awkward silence. *No, no, no.* My stomach flipped. Seconds ticked by, my brain scrambling to break the tension. Horrified, I came up empty. Just like that, my perfect evening was tarnished.

Tony picked up his train of thought. I stewed with mine.

Theo could be gruff, no doubt. A tad *rough around the edges*, as both my parents had said. At work that gruffness was an asset. He was in charge of telling people—sometimes hundreds of them—what to do and how to do it. Theo had to make people listen and solve problems of enormous scale for a living. His no-nonsense command had swept me off my feet. But at home, with a young daughter, I'd often had to remind Theo that Faith and I weren't stagehands. We didn't work for him. He'd say okay, he knew, he was sorry. "I get it." And do it again anyway.

He didn't have to be so obvious about correcting her. Was a six-year-old supposed to have perfect table manners? And even if Faith *was* rude, it was more a reflection on us than her. This wasn't our first difficult exchange in front of other people. Embarrassing. Why couldn't we get this right? I'd spoken to my therapist about our problematic communication and was a year into graduate school, still clueless about how to defuse this kind of tension.

The girls gobbled up their last bites of food and fled to Faith's room to play. I excused myself to scoop ice cream into the Frankenstein bowls I'd purchased special for the occasion and delivered the creamy goodness to Faith's room. Back in the kitchen, chatting with Evelyn, I kept up my facade—smiling. Everything was fine, thank you. Soon the girls reappeared, empty Frankenstein bowls held out, waiting for more. I started toward the freezer.

"No, that's okay," Evelyn said. "Mia's had enough."

I stopped in my tracks, my chest tight. Something about Evelyn's inflection. The words "no" and "enough." Underneath the words, I heard—or rather, felt—something else. I weighed less than I had in ages, was enjoying a respite from recording my food every day in a tracker, but I imagined she meant to add, "And so has Faith."

Mia was a wisp of a girl, a tiny little thing. So were her parents. Evelyn's comment was so, well, public. It carried the implication that a good mother says no, a good mother follows through, a good mother denies. I was fucking up. I knew it. Again. Still. Had known it for years. Since the first time the pediatrician had indicated Faith's weight was high, since those failed friendships. I wanted to enjoy myself, and I wanted Faith to enjoy herself too, not only with food but with everything. I wanted her to be free from worry, and I never said no to treats on special nights like Halloween. But Evelyn, whether on purpose or by accident, had shined light on my inadequacies.

"Go get dressed," I said to the girls, more forcefully than I'd intended.

Evelyn went to put the finishing touches on Mia's costume.

Only later, my hands submerged in a sink of sudsy water, did I finally let myself feel the ache in my chest, the rejection. I was wrong to think I could let my guard down. In my mind, I reviewed and replayed the evening: Tony's sideways glance, the set of Evelyn's mouth, their tones of voice, and Theo's too. Oddly, I felt like I'd done something wrong, gotten in trouble. No amount of careful planning, of attention to detail, had avoided fiasco. I thought about talking to Theo, then quickly discarded the idea. Faith seemed fine now, and he'd drunk a lot of beer. I knew he'd tell me to stop focusing on the negative, look at the positive.

Beyond that, talking to someone else didn't enter my mind. Dad, who I'd moved into a nearby apartment, hadn't been feeling well—his heart and a dementia diagnosis. And I'd learned not to try commiserating with Mom about this sort of thing. Too often, in person or through the phone line, I'd seen that look, had heard the dismissiveness. As if my confusion and struggle hadn't mattered. Somehow, she'd redirect our conversations to be about herself, her problems. Of the *You think that's bad? Listen to this* variety. I had never understood that competitiveness.

Reaching out would only make me look needy and selfish. Instead, I set my shoulders, turned on the faucet, and rinsed the dishes.

Thanksgiving

The day had started like any Thanksgiving—Theo preparing a lot of food. He preferred to work alone in the kitchen, and free to focus on Faith, I didn't argue. She was in second grade now, would turn eight in three weeks' time, old enough to really participate in the holidays. Kneeling at the coffee table, surrounded by red, yellow, orange, and brown construction paper, a stapler, and a pair of scissors, she was amassing the parts for three turkey headdresses. A real turkey, stuffing, green bean casserole, and sweet potatoes were roasting in the oven.

Theo took a short break from the kitchen, rewarding himself with another martini and some football. I wanted him to enjoy himself. He'd gotten home from work in the wee morning hours, and, rather than sleep, he dove straight into preparations. After a decade of marriage, after encouraging Theo for years to rest only to be told, "Chores don't do themselves," after offering to help only to be told, "I got it," I'd given up. He had anxiety. I was sure of it, but whenever I said so he'd shrug and tell me to stop being critical.

Faith stood, a piece of brown paper in her hand. "I have to

measure you, Mom," she said, encircling my head. I held the strip in place while she carefully stapled the ends together. Then she stapled paper feathers to the band. "Wanna help?" she asked me.

"That's okay, love. I'm enjoying just watching you."

The three of us had talked about keeping this year's celebration small, easy, and it was a relief. Mom and Bob were home in New Jersey, spending the day with Bob's family. Theo's huge family—four siblings, married, now with fifteen kids among them, and us—was too unwieldy to host in one location. And Dad, who should have been sitting between us on the couch, had died eight months earlier.

Having Dad close those last few years of his life had been a wonderful gift. The time with Faith was irreplaceable. She'd adored her peepaw and he'd refused ever to disappoint her, shuffling his way, often falling, to every school event, invitation, and family function. Until dementia eroded his mind, he hadn't smiled as hard or laughed as much in a long while. Theo had loved and respected my father too, venerated his World War II combat service. But the strain of moving Dad across the country, managing his failing health, seeing a virile, hilarious man disappear in front of our eyes, hearing him struggle to remember my name, and footing most of the bills had taken a toll on us.

Sandwich generation: it has a name for a reason.

Dad couldn't drive. He'd had needs. Faith had had needs. Theo had had needs. Grad school had had requirements. I was squished somewhere in the middle, between everyone, everything. Doctor appointments, grocery store runs, pharmacy pickups, trips to the VA medical center and hospital, and later, the nursing home. School projects, playdates, and Girl Scouts. Class time, reading, writing, and research. Everyone who'd needed something had asked me for it, and I'd never said no.

Theo's work schedule had begun, during that time, to feel more like an excuse than a requirement. "I need help!" I would yell. “Someone has to pay for all of this,” he would counter. We were both right. An impasse. Resentment, hurt, and anger had festered in the space growing between us.

Now, Dad had been dead for eight months, but I was still strung out, bereaved, and impatient. Theo was exhausted. His drinking had been escalating. We were two people who’d reached our limit; we just didn’t know it yet.

Faith, maneuvering scissor blades through paper, cut more feathers. Theo, splayed out in his favorite chair, looked exhausted.

“You should take a nap,” I said.

“Too much to do,” he said.

Football. Arts and crafts. Holiday food. I thought about how Dad would be enjoying himself, how much I missed him. I sipped my wine, waiting for the ache to dull. Turned my attention back to Faith. “Those are looking great, babe,” I said.

Another strip of brown paper. “Your turn, Dad,” Faith said, stapler in hand.

The three of us, feathers akimbo, looked adorable, regal in a papery way, and I laughed.

“Let’s take some pictures,” I said.

Theo hopped up, dragged together chairs. I got the tripod. We cheesed it up, paper feathers pointing every which way.

My stomach rumbled. “I’m hungry,” I said. “When the hell will we finally eat?”

Theo scowled and I realized, too late, that my attempt at good-natured ribbing had fallen flat. He was too tired, too lubricated, too sensitive. He headed to the kitchen. Cookware banged. Utensils slammed. This was not our first conflict at the juncture of fatigue, misunderstanding, and too much alcohol.

In retrospect, I wish at this exact moment I had kept my mouth shut. I wish I’d given Theo credit for his hard work and conscientiousness. I wish I’d laughed at our silly selves, getting all worked up over nothing. Ignored his overblown reaction. But I didn't stop and neither did he.

I followed him into the kitchen, where I saw what that morning had been a new bottle of vodka was now more than half empty.

"It's Thanksgiving," I hissed. "Can you stop being a jerk?"

"I do all the fucking work," he seethed.

"You WANT to do all the work!" I yelled. "According to you, no one else does anything right." My ears were ringing by then, and I could only pick out certain words he said: ". . . fuck . . . holiday . . . asshole . . ."

A vein stuck out on Theo's forehead. I knew what that meant. I'd seen it before, and there was no way, on Thanksgiving, I'd submit my daughter or myself to his alcohol-fueled ravings.

"Faith," I called, snatching the car keys from the hook. "Let's go."

She obeyed without question, and we rushed toward the front door. I was almost there when Theo grabbed my arm, pinning me against the wall.

"You're not going anywhere." His breath was hot on my cheek, his face menacing. Behind him, light flooded the kitchen, double ovens whirred, cookware covered the counters.

"Yes, we are," I grunted, wrenching myself free. "I'm sick of your bullshit."

I pushed past him toward the car, where Faith waited by the back seat door. I strapped her into the booster seat. "Everything's okay," I said, inanely, kissing her cheek. She just stared at me.

As I tore out of the driveway, Theo watched from the door. In the middle of the cul-de-sac, I punched the gas. Tires screeched.

"Everything's fine, babe," I said again, looking in the rearview mirror. Her blue eyes looked shocked; she remained silent. *Make this okay.* "We're just going on an adventure."

Inside, I was boiling. I didn't want this, to be the person

whisking my daughter away from home on a holiday. I knew deep down Theo didn't want it either.

What was Faith's young mind making of this disaster? The thought to move that query from my brain to my mouth never materialized. An adventure. Somehow that made sense to me, and it was certainly easier than admitting the entire situation was not okay, and having to deal with the result.

On the way to Denny's—where the two of us would eat a dry turkey dinner and kill time until Theo would for sure be passed out—I spotted one or two more cars. I remembered the way Theo had crowed that time he'd quit alcohol for a while. "See," he'd said. "I don't have a problem. You're the one with the problem."

My holier-than-thou response: "At least I don't have beer for breakfast." But since Dad had died, I *was* drinking more than before. I'd have to cut back too.

I pulled into the parking lot, Denny's yellow sign ablaze. Cut the engine. The time had come. Theo had to pick: us or the booze.

"Faith's been talking about Thanksgiving," her teacher said, the following week. I was in the second-grade classroom, preparing to lead a Girl Scout troop meeting.

"Yeah, it wasn't very good," I replied, a fist crushing my heart. I'd told Theo that I would leave him unless he quit drinking. He'd begged me not to break our family up, was researching twelve-step meetings.

"She's telling the other kids and parents how mad her dad was. That the day was bad."

"Thanks for telling me," I said, forcing myself to look her in the eye. In five minutes, twelve little girls, including Faith, would be watching my every move.

Later, at home, I knelt down on the hard hallway floor, taking Faith's hands in mine. "I know Thanksgiving was really hard and scary, sweetheart," I said. Theo, looking sad, sat in the living room, watching us. "I get it, and you can talk to me or Dad any time you want to. But other kids and their parents, they don't know what to do. You talk to us, okay? Not them."

"Okay, Mom," she said, dejected.

I didn't need any graduate-level psychology classes to know I'd just told my daughter that looking fine to other people mattered more than reality.

Girl Scouts

At the front of our local Whole Foods Market, I watched my Brownie Girl Scouts settle around tables. Eleven third-grade girls, plus Faith, for an even dozen. We'd toured the facility with the manager, who'd spoken about where food comes from and concepts like organic farming and sustainability—heady topics for the average eight- or nine-year-old. But the nut butter aisle, with its mechanized dispensers, made up for all that. At the tug of a lever, a ribbon of blended gold expelled into a container, and now, to everyone's delight, a store associate was delivering containers of nut butter, fresh fruit, and crackers to us, seated at the front of the store—life was good. I was chatting with one of the moms, until I turned to smile at Faith. There she was, using a cracker to scoop up a big glob of peanut butter and gobble it down. Then, in rapid succession, she grabbed another and another. I'd never seen this behavior before.

None of the other girls, munching slowly, noticed. I didn't want to embarrass Faith by calling attention to it. But two of the chaperone moms did notice. The two were friends, and I often saw them jogging together, two twigs with legs. Camila, the first mom, leaned in and whispered something to the other mom—whatever her name was—who at least had the decency to look uncomfortable. I already felt self-conscious in a place where every employee looked as if they'd just walked off the set of an REI commercial: fresh-faced, slim, veritably sun-kissed. I radiated mom vibes in Faith's direction, hoping to give her some kind of *cool-it* signal, but she never looked up.

Camila's waifish daughter, like Evelyn's Mia, had been one of my scouts since the beginning, and throughout kindergarten into first grade, we'd frequently swapped our girls for playdates, on rare occasions hanging out together while they played. But Camila's family was angular, of the *always on the go* variety: hiking, biking, running, walking, jumping, skipping, hopping, every –ing imaginable. My family less so. It had seemed like a nice balance, or so I'd thought. But as time had passed, I'd felt Camila pull away. Soon, the girls, too, grew less close.

I'd tried to be good, cheerful. Tried to anticipate whatever I thought folks wanted from me, to make myself the type of person other people liked. I was the mom who made the best snacks for sports, who had the most holiday decorations, and who bought gifts for people, just because. I did not get why my best efforts always backfired. After the cooling off, I'd tried to see the change between the kids as normal, different interests with friends to match, but deep down, I'd worried we'd been judged, that a comparison had been made—mothers may have pretended otherwise, but comparing, both implied and outright, was the norm—and we'd come up short. Again.

I stared hard at Camila. *Bitch. How dare you?* Both of those colluding women were adults who'd taken part in our troop anti-bullying conversations. Awful behavior to model around a group of third graders, but I stood there, polite and silently fuming.

My degree, conferred six months prior to this, sat on a shelf at home, collecting dust. Three years, tens of thousands of dollars, and all that education had not cured my inability to speak up, to handle sensitive interactions or Camila's rudeness. At least Theo was doing better, working the twelve steps and sober since that previous terrible Thanksgiving.

Finally, with snack time reduced to crumbs and dirty faces, we headed home. In the car, Faith thanked me for taking the troop on a field trip. Her hair, which I'd made the mistake in preschool of suggesting we cut into a short pixie (which had looked absolutely adorable, until she came home crying because a boy had said she looked like him), had grown long enough again for pigtails. They sprang from the sides of her head, *swishing* as she spoke. "That was fun! Thanks, Mom!" *Swish*.

"Great, and you're so welcome," I said. "What was your favorite part?"

"The snacks." *Swish*.

I smiled, in spite of myself. Why shouldn't snacks be the favorite? I wanted Faith to enjoy food, not be controlled or upset by it like I was. I didn't want her to feel ashamed for being hungry, for wanting more. I knew that feeling. I saw in it the ghost of my younger self during the time I'd kept sweet snacks secretly stashed in the living room cupboard under the TV. If Mom had ever found them and confronted me, after my guts finished liquefying, I would have simply said I was hungry. What else would a kid say?

As Faith chatted on about the tour, I *hmmm'd* and *huh'd*, wondering whether I should say anything about the way she'd eaten. But each thought sounded more accusatory than the last. *So, babe, why did you do that? Did you see anyone else doing that?* I remembered that time I'd ripped an extra slice of cheese out of her little hand, imperiously tossing it in the trash. Inside, I groaned—one mothering mistake after another.

Resolve gathered in my chest. Over the past year, I had, at long last, been quietly instituting stricter food rules: no seconds, no ice cream, no junk food in the house. For her and for me. Four years after the pediatrician's first comment that Faith's weight was too high, I'd followed through. Faith had on occasion balked, but I'd remained stalwart. It was good for both of us. Her weight had evened out with her growth, but now I was struggling to keep off the fifty pounds I'd lost when she was a baby. Maybe this day's behavior, a rare moment of food-related freedom, was a reaction to heaps of denials.

And, I admitted to myself, if Faith and I had been at home, I, too, would have wolfed down a few goo-globbed crackers. I made my final decision. I'd say nothing about the peanut butter. I'd assume those few minutes were an anomaly.

Bedtime

Faith and I were in her room. Now twelve years old, she still liked to spoon before falling asleep. From the wallpaper, Noah with his animals watched Faith reach for her favorite well-loved stuffed lion, Cherry Puller, bought for her by my mom. The motion, her sleeve riding up, exposed a scratch on her wrist, not deep but about three inches long. It looked intentional.

"What's that?" I said, shocked.

"Nothing," she said. "It's no big deal."

I didn't want to overreact, my brain racing for wisdom. Faith placed her glasses on the dresser, climbed into bed, and scooted over to make room for me. I put my glasses on the dresser, cuddled up next to her. The back of her head, her hair, was by my nose. I smelled floral shampoo, chlorine. "Dad and I love you so much." *That's all I've got?* "Life would never be the same if anything happened to you," I added.

"I know," she said, settling in.

I tightened my hug. "By the way, have I told you lately that I love you?"

This was our game, and she always said no.

"No."

I followed up with my standard line. "I love you to the moon and back."

THUNK

It was late September, two months after my mom died and a month after Faith started eighth grade, when Dr. Kay had first said that Faith needed help. For several days afterward, I vetted names from the list she'd sent me, left messages. Finding a therapist who was accepting new adolescent patients and had less than a two-month-long waiting list was proving difficult. I made calls and waited, made more calls and waited.

I was also planning Mom's ash commitment ceremony. Bob was due to arrive soon, so I contacted a boat company, reviewed catering options, and alerted family and friends. Faith now refused to eat out, so we stopped frequenting restaurants. In the kitchen, while Theo or I cooked, she would shadow us, keeping an eye on our preparations. If we reached for the olive oil, she'd say, "Fat makes you fat." If we reached for the salt, she'd say, "Salt makes you retain water." She forbade any ingredient she considered unhealthy. Ketchup? No. Barbeque sauce? Nope. Butter? Forget it. We ate our bland meals in front of the TV, watching Food Network, and if we changed the channel, she changed it right back.

"Maybe watching will make her hungry," I said to Theo.

Faith, sitting on the floor, her plate on the coffee table, stared at the screen, rarely moving the fork to her mouth. Theo would say, "Honey, you have to eat some more." Or, "Okay, you've got our attention." Faith's most common retort was to tell us to leave her alone, that she was fine. "You're the ones with the problem," she'd say.

At the end of September, an eating disorder specialist named Mona returned my message. Over the phone, I sketched out the basic details regarding Faith, and we scheduled an introductory appointment for Theo and me for the following week, the first week of October.

But first, on the day of Faith's next dance class, I picked her up from school and drove straight home. "I told you this morning," I said, opening the front door, "if I didn't see you eat breakfast, you couldn't dance."

Faith stormed in behind me. "I'm going to that class!" she screamed.

She chucked her backpack across the kitchen, stomped down the hall, and slammed her bedroom door. Noises erupted from the direction of her room. A grunt. A yell.

I grabbed Finn, our cat, and sank into the couch. Too on edge to sit still, I put Finn down, paced the living room. *Bang*. What the hell was she doing in there? I was afraid of her rage, but I set my shoulders and opened her door anyway. One of her heavy boots lay on the floor by the window, blinds askew.

"GET OUT!" she screamed.

I gripped the doorknob. "Faith—"

"Leave me alone. I hate you. This is all your fault. You let me get fat."

My brain had no time to register the pain and the truth of her words.

"I'm such a fat ass," she wailed. "Everyone is half my size."

I moved toward the edge of her bed, where she sat, wanting to offer her a hug, sit next to her—anything. But she sank to the floor, arched her back, and bashed her forehead into the thick wooden frame of her bed. *Thunk*. Her head rebounded back, her eyes closed. She screamed like a wild animal.

I raced toward her, fell to my knees. "Babe, please." I protected her head with my hand to cushion the next blow. "Please, stop!" She threw her head forward again, smashing my hand.

I tried to hug her, but she pushed hard against me, her muscles like stone. I scrambled back up to put my body between her and the bed frame.

She tried to keep up the fight but finally sat back. Tears slid down her cheeks, and she collapsed into my lap.

"It's so hard," she sobbed into my stomach. "Why does it have to be so hard?"

I rubbed her back, fighting tears of my own. "I don't know, sweetheart."

She wrapped her arms around me. *My sweet, sweet sensitive girl*. I stroked her forehead. No lump yet and nothing Boo-Boo Kitty could heal, anyway. I tried to summon something, anything from the memory banks of my grad school practicum, but what words could possibly help this kind of pain, this level of anguish?

Should haves raced through my mind. I should have banned sugar, all white foods for that matter. I should have pretended to love exercise. I should have made a bigger deal out of the lie of perfection we watched every day on TV. I wanted to demolish every kid, every bully who'd ever hurt her feelings or made fun of her, every adult too. I wanted to smash the television. What right did the world have to make my thirteen-year-old daughter feel like she was less than enough? I wanted to take her and escape, but there was nowhere to go.

Faith sat up, wiping her eyes. Mascara smudged her cheeks. "I have to go to the bathroom."

I stayed on the floor in a stupor. Her words from minutes earlier rang in my ears: *It's your fault. I hate you*. And she was right.

I had failed her. I stared at my soggy mascara-smudged jeans, noticed the roundness of my stomach. Felt the fullness of my hips and thighs. Back in size 14s. Jesus. I couldn't keep my shit together, for me or her. My body was the one Faith knew most intimately besides her own. It was *my* body she saw every day and over time contracting, expanding. Me she watched in front of the mirror. I wondered if the outline she saw when she looked in the mirror was mine.

A multitude of Noahs' eyes bored into me from every direction, and I felt exposed. To my right, a small hot-pink plastic baby doll crib overflowed with stuffed animals, the baby doll long since given away or forgotten somewhere. Cherry Puller, Faith's favorite lion, sat on top of the heap, king of the jungle. His fur, once plush and fluffy, was nubby and worn from the hours he'd spent in her arms. He was tipped to one side, surveying his kingdom. I must have been a sorry sight. To my left, the other boot Faith had been wearing lay where she'd thrown it, next to her bookcase. Shelves packed with the Warrior series cat books she'd been obsessed with during the transition from elementary to middle school. I'd hoofed it to our local Borders' going-out-of-business sale to snatch every available volume, barely able to carry them all.

She'd loved to position herself on the couch between our real cats at the time, Randall and Little Kitty, to read to them. I remembered the huge pile of Warrior drawings she'd made—cats, with names from the books like Firestar and Graystripe, prowling at night in the deep, dark wood. How I'd relished watching her, hunched over the coffee table, surrounded by a rainbow of pencils, pens, markers, and crayons. So intent, determined to capture the fantasies at play in her imagination. Sometimes she'd crafted stories of her own with the books' characters, and I'd listened, enthralled, yearning for ingenuity like hers.

But hitting her head like that. *There's more to this than me.* My pep talk sounded insincere. Realizing she was still in the bathroom, I hoisted myself off the floor, walked to the closed door. A light pink glow, from the paint, shined from under the door. "You okay in there?"

She said she was, and I figured she wanted to be alone. I headed toward the kitchen. Dinner still had to be prepared whether or not anyone felt like eating.

I pulled the salad ingredients and a bottle of white wine out of the fridge. Poured myself a glass. Theo had quit drinking but didn't mind that I still did. I stood over the cutting board chopping a cucumber, sipping. I heard Faith leave her bathroom. My heart ached knowing how much pain she was in. I grabbed a tomato. Salad was a zero-point food on the Weight Watchers plan. Having one at the ready made me feel like I was doing my job as a mom.

I took another swig of wine, sighed. I tilted my head from side to side, drew my shoulder back trying to release the throbbing pain I now noticed under my right blade. Out the kitchen window, beyond the houses across the street, past the neighbor's palm trees, Boney Peak, our mountain. *Just a big hill*, some might say. Either way, to me: majestic. Soon Bob would be here, people would be in the house to celebrate Mom. Would we get through it without a scene? There was no way to know. I ripped a couple of celery stalks from the bunch, punched the knife blade down, each blow thumping against the cutting board.

1973

One day, Dad, who'd moved back home, said, "Let's go."

We escaped out the front door toward the carport and Mom's bright red car. She stayed behind, like usual. She didn't care about our adventures. Too bad for her!

"M'lady," Dad said, bowing next to the open car door.

I scrambled in, my shoes squeaking against slick red leather. Inside smelled a lot like the place where we went to buy my special shoes, the ones with cookies because my feet were flat. My feet looked normal to me, but the idea of cookies in my shoes made me laugh. I was five years old.

Dad checked the rearview mirror, cranked his window down. I cranked mine down too. I usually did whatever Dad did. If he wore a tie, I wore one too. If he whistled, I whistled too, except I couldn't really whistle so it sounded like air blowing out of my mouth. If he played the piano, I plunked the keys. If he pulled out his drawing pad, I asked for a pencil. Dad always said yes. It was him and me against the world, especially when Mom was in what Dad called *one of her moods*. Which she was a lot. Sometimes she'd ask me what my problem was. Usually, I wasn't sure what she meant. But I sure wondered what her problem was. Why she'd rather be alone than with me and Dad.

The engine rumbled to life. "We're off!" Dad said.

I didn't know where we were going, and it didn't matter. The only thing that mattered was we were together. We passed the neighbor's house, and I caught a whiff of Dad's spicy cologne. He smelled good.

Dad pointed to the pile of 8-track cassettes on the floor. "Pick one."

As we pulled onto the highway, wind whipped my hair, stinging my face and tickling my ear. I shoved a cassette into the player, and Dad cranked up the volume. "*And they called it puppy looooovvvvveeeeee*," soared out of the speakers. Dad smiled at me, and he was happy, so I was happy. The front seat was like a couch, nothing between us, so I cozied up next to him.

Together, we barreled down the road.

THE FIX

Theo and I sat on the couch across from Mona. Long curly blond hair, perfectly coifed, surrounded her face like a dewy waterfall, and her smile offered calm assurance that she knew what she was doing. I felt an overwhelming sense of relief. Mona was the fix we needed.

Worry rushed out of me in a torrent of words as I explained: two and half months since Mom's unexpected death, Faith's weight loss, her emotional volatility, and the addendum of the head-banging incident. Theo might have said something had I given him the chance. Instead, he listened to my recitation without facial expression or commentary. At home, we debated what to do and why, but in public, his behavior was different. His worry manifested as stoicism.

Mona nodded, like she'd heard our story before. I said nothing about my degree. I was too ashamed. "What did we do wrong?" I asked Mona, breathless.

"It's normal to feel guilty and responsible, but neither of you did anything wrong," she said. "That line of thinking won't do you any good."

She handed me a stack of paperwork and delivered her speech with surgical precision. Mona explained that eating disorders weren't an attempt to get attention. I glanced at Theo. Eating disorders, she said, were an unhealthy attempt to change low self-esteem. Faith was terrified of not measuring up, and this was her mind's way of coping with fear and anger toward herself. "You absolutely must not get into any more power struggles around food."

On my paper I wrote, *NO power struggle.* I knew what she meant. The house felt like a war zone. Every mealtime, my chest tightened with anxiety. Faith approached from the flank, wary, prepared to defend her position. Each bite was a battle of wills. She wanted the power to control her body. I wanted the power my position as her mother was supposed to afford me. That is, I wanted her to listen, obey, eat. Live. One of us had to wave the white flag now, and apparently it would have to be me. While the first therapy I'd had hadn't fixed me, it had helped me feel better. Dolly, my therapist, had heard me. She'd held space for me. She'd helped me see I could question my own thoughts, their validity. And we'd talked about positive coping mechanisms like healthy food, exercise, and journal writing. That's what Faith needed, too, ways to cope with life's vagaries.

I would trust this process. I would watch Faith throw away or ignore her food, listen to her berate herself, fear another breakdown, and try not to do a goddamn thing to intervene. Act as normal as possible. Could I do it?

"I'd better get started with her ASAP," Mona said. "I'll see her twice a week, until I get a better understanding of what's going on."

Mona explained her fee structure and that she didn't bill insurance. Theo made a low "whoa" sound, and I did some quick mental math—a hefty sum. Mona added that Faith would also need to see a nutritionist every week. Even with health insurance, a large chunk of our monthly income would be needed to pay for treatment, and I realized that in the near future I might have to return to work. But for now, I earmarked the life insurance money from

Mom's death. I would pay a thousand dollars a session, for as long as possible, if it meant Faith would get better.

Mona suggested a consultation with a psychiatrist for psychotropic medication. Simultaneously, Theo and I said, "No."

We stood. "By the way," Mona said, "don't forget to prioritize your relationship. This can be a rocky road."

At home, Theo went to the garage to tinker and decompress. I carried Mona's paperwork toward the couch. A picture on the mantel caught my eye: Mom and Bob, plus Theo, Faith—just shy of her sixth birthday—and me on vacation in Hawaii, an all-time favorite.

I leaned in close. The five of us were dressed in the same bright red fabric with a repeating pattern of giant white hibiscus flowers. God, how nerdy I'd felt, walking around the hotel in matching outfits, snapping photos on the lawn, even though it was my idea. That trip had always stood out to me as a grandmothering home run. Every morning, Mom wrapped bread in a napkin at breakfast so she and Faith could feed the swans on the property pond. Faith hadn't grown up next to a lake the way I had. Mom held her hand as they approached the pond, tenderly teaching Faith to crouch down and be careful. "Don't startle them. Hold the bread, just so." Side by side, they squatted at the water's edge, waiting patiently for the swans to float up. Even from a distance, I could sense Faith holding her breath.

To a kid, swans are huge, and I knew they could also be mean. Faith copied Grandma's every move, her hand extended until a swan neared, craned its neck, and plucked the bread right from Faith's fingers. Afterward, her eyes wide as saucers, she called, "Mommy, did you see that?" Mom had chosen a luau with hula lessons, cheering when Faith joined in, and, because of the six-hour New Jersey to Hawaii time difference, took Faith on early morning beach excursions to watch the sun's rays wake the sky. *Now, never again.*

I sank into the couch, Mona's papers in my lap. Information still seemed like the key to calming the quiver in my chest. If I could learn enough about what was happening with Faith, I'd know how to fix it. Or at least not make it worse.

I read about what eating disorders were not: diets gone out of control, deceitful vanity, anyone's fault, or a way to get back at people. I made a mental note to bring that up with Theo, who kept asking me why Faith was doing this to us. I never admitted to Theo that I felt that way sometimes, too, before quickly releasing the notion. No way was *Hurt Mom and Dad* foremost in Faith's mind. She had an illness. The literature said Theo and I were to regulate Faith's schedule, keep meals predictable, and give her advanced notice of plans to eat out. Easy. We weren't eating out anymore. We were to encourage her to cope with feelings by writing them down, and we were allowed to offer unconditional positive regard.

My thoughts volleyed back and forth. Theo and I had always praised Faith's efforts, commended a job well done. We told her every day how much we loved her. "Have I told you lately that I love you?" Our game. How many times had I said it? And, yes. Our issues, those periods of time when life, our parenting, had been less than stellar. But all families have history. We were as normal, as ordinary as anyone else. Mona had said not to worry about why this was happening. Still, how could I not?

What most surprised me about the information was the similarity to some of what I'd learned about overeating in the many diet programs I'd tried. Eating disorders numbed feelings and fulfilled a need for distraction: same as overeating. How many times, feeling sad or unhappy, had I sat on the couch to mindlessly watch hours of television while chowing down a burger and fries? I never imagined that *not* eating could do the same thing.

Scanning the paper, my eyes returned to the same two points: eating disorders are an unhealthy attempt to change low self-esteem, and they are a coping mechanism for being terrified of not measuring up. But what I wanted to know, what I never could know, was the amount of cause and effect: nature versus nurture. In the future, I will wonder why this same rubric was never applied to me, my relationship with food, myself, or my years of yo-yo dieting, but the cultural value will be painfully obvious: fat people are just fat and lazy, while thin people warrant concern and care.

Now, on the couch, I only wondered if Mona had peeked into my heart to create this list.

The next morning, Faith walked into the kitchen, yawning. On the counter, the bag of egg bagels I'd purchased in a spurt of optimism. Theo and I had informed Faith of her therapy appointment, and we hoped that would be the evidence she needed to understand this was serious. And maybe it was. Her demeanor was soft. I felt no antagonism. She didn't look angry or like she wanted to pick a fight. I took a small breath. My words needed to sound just right.

"I bought bagels," I said. Perfect. I didn't sound desperate or pleading or demanding. I sounded, well, normal. How I used to sound before.

"Okay," she said.

Oh, my god. She said yes. Yes!

"Great," I said, nonchalant.

I grabbed the bag, shoved a bagel into the toaster, and yanked the strawberry cream cheese out of the fridge. I wanted to get the food in front of her before she had the chance to change her mind. The toaster popped, I smeared the bagel, threw it onto her plate. I sat, too, tried not to stare, not to look like our fate rested upon this bagel.

She took a bite. I held my breath. I waited. She swallowed. She smiled.

She smiled!

I hadn't realized how much I'd missed her beautiful braces. And that smile! It had been so long. She took another bite. I could have sworn she looked relieved. My plan was already working. And just like that, the worry, anger, and fear of the last couple of months dissolved.

"It's good, right?"

She nodded. I took a sip of coffee, relaxed into my chair.

I knew we had a long way to go but figured this was a major step in the right direction. Faith was eating! She seemed to like it! She smiled! I didn't want her to feel like a specimen under a microscope, so I stared into my coffee cup.

A few minutes later, Faith finished her bagel, even downed her gummy vitamins regardless of the fifteen calories! She washed it all down with a little bit of orange juice.

"Phew," she said. "I'm full."

I bet. Her stomach had probably shrunk to the size of a walnut from lack of use. But I bit my lip, afraid any comment might be taken as confirmation that she'd overeaten. I took her plate to the sink.

"Thanks, Mom," she said, standing up.

She said thanks!

"Welcome, babe."

We'd had thousands of pleasant exchanges like this, but now I couldn't remember the last one.

"Mom, I really don't think I need Mona. I'm feeling a lot better."

"I am *so* glad, sweetheart, but I think we need to stick with the plan, at least for a while until we see how you're doing."

She looked like she wanted to disagree, but said nothing. She headed to her room.

I couldn't help myself. *We're going to be the lucky ones.* The ones who got this licked early. I was sure of it. I grabbed the loaf of 100% whole wheat bread, the all-natural peanut butter, and the organic grape jelly and set about making Faith's favorite sandwich. For the first time in a long time, I thought it might not end up in the middle school trash can.

Marie and I had met in grad school, and when I scheduled a lunch date with her soon after Faith ate the bagel, what I mostly wanted was to pick her smart brain. The bagel hadn't solved our problem, and I needed a therapist for myself, a fix for myself, someone with whom I could freely and safely share my thoughts and feelings about what was happening.

Marie was a true wonder. Back in school, we'd bonded over hours of class time, exam study, and a running joke. After about the third time we both earned As for papers on the same topic—hers at eight pages and mine at twenty—I started saying, "Why make it easy when it can be way harder?" She'd chuckle, shrug. Never did I figure out how to cram twenty pages' worth of information into eight, like Marie. She'd been a kind face when Dad had died, had babysat back then for Faith, and was fond of Theo. I'd even invited her to join my book club.

After graduation, I'd decided against becoming a therapist—too many additional training hours to complete, too many unhappy people in the world, and too little pay for such important, draining work. Marie, however, had stuck with it and was now interning with a group of licensed clinicians. I knew she wouldn't judge me, and I trusted her to keep my confidence. No other family or friends knew yet about Faith's eating disorder. No one else seemed to have this sort of problem. I was embarrassed and ashamed of my inadequacies. Five years had passed since graduation, but I still believed that the training should have enabled me to protect my daughter.

The day of our lunch date, Marie came to the house. We hugged hello, headed for the couch. Faith was at school. Theo, golfing or on one of the freelance gigs he so often took now that he was retired.

"How are things?" Marie wanted to know.

"Honestly, a little rough right now." Tears threatened. I clenched my shoulder muscles, willed myself not to cry. I despised this weakness in myself. "We're having some trouble with Faith—it's an eating disorder. It's been really hard since my mom died." *Keep it together.*

Marie wrapped her arms around me. "I'm so sorry."

"Thanks," I said, stiffening. "I just—"

I just what? The living room closed in on me. How could I put into words what I was feeling about the inadequacies I'd spent my life trying to hide? That even though Theo and I were in this together, I felt totally alone? That every time he wrapped me in his strong arms, reassuring me Faith would be fine, I imagined head-butting him. How nothing I said was helping her. That as much time as the teachers at grad school had spent talking to us about nature, they'd spent as much or more time talking about nurture. That when Mona had said I wasn't to blame, I'd felt more at fault than before.

I cared about Marie, but she wasn't a mom. I didn't think she could understand; I didn't think anyone could. She released my stiff body from the hug, sat back, and waited.

"I need some advice," I finally said.

"Oh, I'm here for you, but let's not do therapy." Indeed, since Marie was my friend, to be my therapist would be a conflict of interest. But I knew the rules.

"I'm not asking you for therapy," I said. "I need a referral, someone great, someone who has experience with these issues." What I didn't add, because I couldn't say it, was that I needed help.

Marie smiled. "I know just the person."

1974

I stood on the stairway landing, a stick from the backyard slung over my shoulder, like how Opie Taylor carried his fishin' pole. A handkerchief with a snack hung off the end. I didn't want to get hungry. I looked down at my parents. They looked up at me—two pairs of blinking eyes. "I'm running away," I said. I was five and a half years old, maybe six.

Mom looked at Dad. Dad looked at me. "Where will you go?" he asked.

Oh. Where would I go? I had no idea. I hadn't thought about that, because I didn't really want to run away. I wanted them to listen to me, pay attention to me, and help me. Why didn't they care how I felt? Was Pennsylvania far? Auntie Anne was my favorite. She always let me sit on her lap and run my fingers through her soft, long brown hair. She always smiled at me, gave me as many hugs as I wanted. She always stroked my face, took such good care of me. I wished Mom would do more of that.

I was still thinking when Dad said, "I need you to know something." He put his hands on his hips. "If you walk out that door, you can never come back."

My stomach sank. My body went squishy. I felt sick, like throw-up sick. Never come back?

Never coming back meant no Bumpy, no canopy, no ice-skating. It meant no Mom and no Dad. Behind them, out the back windows, I could see my lake. I didn't want to never come back. How could Dad say that to me? It was supposed to be me and him against the world. He was always on my side, no matter what Mom said. She might have told me not to come home. But Dad? Nuh-uh. This was her fault. I was sure of it. Just like when he was gone.

I went back to my room, threw the stupid stick, and sat on the floor. Now I was stuck there, miserable. They didn't even ask me why I thought leaving might be better than staying. I didn't matter.

SINKING

Waves gently rocked the boat. Seagulls soared overhead. Mid-October, a glorious fall morning off the Oxnard coast. Warm sun. Crisp breeze. Clear blue sky. A small group of family and friends had joined Bob and me for Mom's commitment ceremony, and the captain had motored us to a location he said was frequented by pods of dolphins. Bob and I stood on the stern, between us a scallop shell–shaped biodegradable container with Mom's ashes. We spoke about Mom, listened to others speak of her—the occasional stench, like rotten eggs, of diesel fuel the morning's only blemish.

Together, Bob and I carried the shell to the side of the boat. Everyone gathered around. Bob and I looked at each other, nodded, and tossed it overboard. *Thwump.* Splash.

One by one, people tossed carnations onto the shell. Sea water, soaking through the biodegradable material, bubbled. Next to me, Faith tossed her flower in too. She made no effort to wipe away the tears streaming down her face. I pulled her into an embrace, and for the first time in a while she didn't flinch or pull away or tell me to leave her alone. She felt more delicate than I was used to.

"Grandma loved you so much, babe," I said, my voice cracking. I didn't know what else to say. Faith nodded.

The shell slipped fully beneath the surface, gliding ever downward, leaving us and the floating array of flowers behind.

I wondered what Faith was thinking about. Was she replaying a slide show of happy memories? Indoor waterslides and real wolves, from that time Mom and Bob took her to the Great Wolf Lodge? The easel and paints Mom set up at her place, just for Faith? Picking fresh zucchinis from the neighbor's garden, standing side by side to make bread together? Or was it the future Faith was envisioning? I tightened my grip around her waist, breaking the spell. She pulled away to go sit with her best friend, Isabelle.

I turned my face to the sun. This day—commitment at sea—was the only instruction I'd gotten from Mom related to death. She was adamant about not being in the ground. The idea had terrified her, and regardless of the complicated anatomy of our relationship, I'd been determined to carry out her wishes. Here and now, my best for once enough.

"Look, over there!" someone called. Dolphins! Zooming around the boat and out from underneath it.

I scanned the spot where the shell had been, still covered with carnations. Dolphins streaming by. "Bye, Mom," I said.

Just then, a flash in my peripheral vision.

A dolphin vaulted out of the water, full arc, twisting. I gasped. Had it understood why we were there? *A sign?*

I turned to my niece. "Did you see that?" I wanted to be sure I hadn't imagined that beautiful sight.

She smiled.

DRAMA QUEEN

Back onshore, Theo, Faith, and I piled into the car. Bob had driven separately, and we'd invited everyone back to the house to continue celebrating Mom.

As Theo pulled out of the marina parking lot, heading toward home, neighborhoods and strip malls gave way to open farmland. Huge fields of dark, rich soil stretched before us in every direction. At harvest time, Oxnard's most common crops include celery, strawberries, lemons, avocados, and leafy greens. Oxnard strawberries are, in fact, famous, and until I moved to Newbury Park, I'd never realized how close to downtown Los Angeles California's vast agricultural landscape reached. Straight ahead, in the distance, stretched a mountain range whose name I didn't know, had never thought to find out. And off to the right, the back side of our beloved Boney Peak.

Staring out the window, rushing past the fertile ground, we were quiet, lost in our own thoughts. In my mind, on repeat: that dolphin jumping out of the water. I believed in the energetic interconnectedness of people, animals, and nature. If we slowed down enough to notice, stuff like that was happening all the time. Right after Mom died, Bob and I were at the funeral parlor making arrangements, and I'd been seated next to a window. The man behind the big, heavy desk had droned on and on about prayer cards, caskets, service options, and costs. I was trying to listen, but I was exhausted, grieving. Suddenly, just beyond the glass, I'd noticed about a dozen butterflies. Maybe more. Orange, yellow, blue, and black. Bright. Right there, floating and fluttering, but not, as butterflies normally would, flying away. They'd remained, hovering, framed by the window.

"Wow," I'd said, interrupting the man mid-sentence.

He'd paused, his gaze following mine. "Huh," he'd said. "Weird. I've never seen them do that."

I'm still with you, I'd taken that sign to mean, same as the dolphin.

Theo made the turn that took us past the back side of California State University Channel Islands, built on property that had once been home to the Camarillo State Mental Hospital. Fascinated by psychiatric ward stories, I'd read that the facility, opened in 1936 and in operation for sixty years, had housed upwards of seven thousand mentally ill and developmentally disabled patients, making it the largest hospital of its kind in the world. But as the years had passed and times changed, the national attitude had shifted toward deinstitutionalization. A dwindling patient population and rising costs had shuttered the doors in 1997. Rather than another strip mall, I was glad the land had been developed for something equally as important and necessary.

For the remaining few minutes of the drive, the calm before another flurry of activity, I turned my thoughts to the near future. Ahead of time, knowing this day on the water would be emotionally challenging, I'd purchased four tickets to see a new show everyone was raving about, *The Book of Mormon*. My love of musical theater predated Faith. As a kid, the only present I'd wanted for birthdays or special occasions was tickets to Broadway, and as often as finances had allowed, my parents complied—Mom my number one companion.

I'd started taking Faith as a toddler to age-appropriate shows, *Sesame Street Live!* and the like. Mom had continued the Broadway trend for Faith with *Beauty and the Beast*. Together, we'd taken her to see *The Lion King*. A steady stream of rising curtains, escalating orchestras, and soaring vocals. Whether Faith's passion for musical theater was fused into her DNA or had grown organically from proximity, I would never know. But I could know that come Tuesday, the house lights would dim, the curtain would rise, the orchestra would play, and we'd both get gooseflesh. My daughter would smile, maybe even laugh. And, if history was any indication, within a week, two at the most, Faith would have memorized the entire soundtrack. I could only hope that once again, in the near future, random bursts of song would resound down the hallway.

It had become Theo's most common comment: "I miss Faith's singing."

"Is Faith okay?" Bob asked me.

He'd been staying with us, and it had been impossible to fully hide Faith's struggle. I'd made excuses of one kind or another for the tears, for why she'd only eat in her room, but it was obvious something significant was going on. The tension was palpable.

"She's having a hard time," I said. "Don't worry. We're working on it."

He looked like he wanted more details. He had known Faith since birth, was her beloved uncle Bob, but I added nothing. I felt ashamed of myself, and I couldn't talk now about Faith without crying. He let the matter drop.

Dinnertime. Bob and Theo were in the kitchen. Faith and I were in her room. I sat on the bed, she sat at her desk, a dinner plate in front of her with goat cheese, lentils, and brown rice rolled in Swiss chard—a Faith-approved dish that I'd prepared at her request, gone cold. The warmer feelings from Mom's commitment ceremony had dissipated, and I'd been gently coaxing Faith to eat for what? An hour? Longer? I could see the struggle on her face—the desire and the hate, the need and the disgust. She picked up her fork, speared a small amount of food, and stared at it.

The door burst open. Theo. Before I could stop him, he yelled at Faith, "Stop acting like such a drama queen!"

"No, you don't—" Faith squeaked. That was as far as she could go. She dropped the fork, hung her head.

"Faith, you need to just get over this and find something to be happy about," he said.

"Get the hell out of here," I seethed.

He hesitated, staring at us before slamming the door.

Find something to be happy about—if he said that one more time . . . If people could just *get over* whatever was wrong, they would! No one would have a single issue! That was not how life worked. I imagined this was Theo's childhood talking, the method his parents had deployed to "help him" with his problems.

More than once over the years, and without sensitivity, I'd told Theo to just *get over* his abrupt communication style. I knew that underneath his alpha male exterior, underneath the way he'd learned to communicate, he cared deeply about us, Faith's pain, this illness, what was happening, and what we could or should do to help. I'd seen it, and it's unfair that my memory can't define or construct more moments here that show Theo's front-facing softer side. But about the Theo of this time period, his future self agrees: soft was rare. He was as scared and confused as I was. As powerless, which made him defensive. He'd spent his entire career fixing problems. His favorite line about anything broken: "I won't quit until I figure out what's wrong with it." His inability to fix this problem fueled his sense of inadequacy, same as it did for me.

Who knew what had prompted this particular outburst? Perhaps, in my absence, Bob had questioned him; perhaps he'd made a comment. Maybe Theo had felt cornered, afraid of saying the wrong thing, of what I would do if I found out. He had reason to be concerned. I always let him know when I thought he'd made a mistake. Clearly, he was impatient and annoyed. We both were. Every meal was punctuated by major disruption. But I was livid, because the pain from what he'd said was evident in Faith's demoralized face, her deflated body.

PENDULUMS

I pushed the button next to the nameplate: Kim P. A few minutes later, I was following her down a hallway and into her office. Small. Cozy. Smelled good. It felt like a safe cocoon. Kim was the therapist Marie had recommended for me to work with one-on-one, and this was our first meeting, early November.

Kim's smile was warm like Mona's. I liked what it did to her eyes. "How can I help?" she asked.

"It's my daughter," I said, the floodgates opening. Kim pointed to the tissue box.

I regurgitated the story, ending with the newest pieces of information. That after Faith ate the bagel she had started eating more, but sometimes she couldn't stop. Then she'd refuse for a while to eat anything, then overeat, again. Mona had called it the pendulum effect. And after the most recent swim practice, Faith had come home crying, raging, and wailing about what a terrible swimmer she was. She'd dropped onto the kitchen floor, slapping herself about the head.

"Sometimes I feel like *I'm* losing my mind," I said. "I can't do this by myself."

"You don't have to," Kim said.

Our first fifty minutes came to an end, and I mentioned our mutual friend, Marie, leaving out the part about how we met.

Kim handed me the standard packet of paperwork. "Remember," she said, "Faith wants to see you taking care of yourself."

"I'm sorry?" I stared at her, unable to parse the sentence.

"Faith wants to know you're doing okay."

I doubted Faith was thinking about me, and I didn't want her to. And the idea that Kim's suggestion to take care of myself was exactly what I wanted Faith to do never occurred to me. Instead, I wondered how a mother could take care of herself while her child languished. What kind of mother *would* take care of herself while her child languished?

The time for taking care of myself, when it might have made a difference, had passed. Since Mom's death and worse since Faith's diagnosis, I wasn't exercising, and I ate healthy meals but only because I was preparing them for Faith. I was eating too much, like I always did when stressed. Every day, I slipped on sweatpants, put my hair in a clip. It didn't matter how I felt or looked—nothing mattered but helping Faith get well.

She's right, you know.

I was in my bathroom, the next morning, staring at the sweatpants I'd draped over the side of the tub. Kim's words about taking care of myself had been stuck on repeat in my mind. I did need to take better care of myself. I was trying, I was always trying, I argued with myself.

On days that required me to look and behave normally, I did. I had dressed up for Mom's commitment ceremony, to go to *The Book of Mormon*, and for my recent doctor appointment. Terrified by Mom's stroke and the heart attack that had actually killed her, I'd gone to see my primary care doctor, filling her in. Mom was only sixty-seven years old, had had no obvious signs or symptoms of heart disease. Bob and I had not understood what went wrong, how she could have improved enough to receive physical and occupational therapy at the rehab center only to end up dead. And we never would understand.

The death certificate had shed no new light, listing as the cause an anterior wall myocardial infarction. Fancy words for heart attack. In search of information, an explanation that made sense, Bob and I had called various doctors involved in Mom's care. Each response had been the same, a form of "We're so sorry, but these things just happen."

My aunt—scientist, Mensa member, and executive in pharmaceuticals—had provided me with the only clue. She'd said that Mom had had high cholesterol for years. I'd had no idea. She never mentioned it to me. My aunt had gone on to say that Mom had tried standard treatment with a statin but had hated the side effects, opting instead for a holistic approach. Clear as day, her grimace-y mouth and raised eyebrows had read, *Bad idea*.

My doctor had ordered blood work, even an echocardiogram since it turned out that both of my parents had had heart disease. Other than needing to lose some weight, I'd received an excellent bill of health. Same as always. But I'd done more than that to take care of myself. I'd gotten a massage and a facial. I'd gone as planned to my recent book club gathering, where I'd chatted, smiled, and thanked everyone for their kind words about my mom, leaving out anything about Faith. I'd started therapy with Kim, planned the following week to have breakfast with Isabelle's mom, and go to a baby shower. Plenty of activities that implied good caretaking, healthy self-prioritization.

But inside, my emotions were riding their own pendulum: rage to despair, desperation to worry. Back and forth. My guts quivered, the front part of my throat ached, and that spot under my right shoulder blade now throbbed constantly. Around this time, Mona alerted us that she was amending Faith's original diagnosis of an eating disorder (which was not anorexia but eating disorder, not otherwise specified, or NOS) to include a second diagnosis of severe depression. So in between scouring cookbooks and the internet for recipes, cooking meals I hoped would keep Faith calm, weighing and measuring her food to the nutritionist's specifications, driving her to and from appointments, and reading books about eating disorders, I searched for books about depression too.

And on those mornings, when I stared at my sweatpants hanging on the side of the tub, I tried to muster the energy for a different choice, but I'd slide the soft cotton over my skin, put that clip in my hair, and start the day.

Faith's behaviors and emotions kept swinging back and forth. Theo, on the other hand, remained in a constant state of high alert, pegged to the red zone. We no longer discussed anything but Faith's illness and what might happen next. Sometimes I avoided his hugs. We rarely kissed. The night his hand had reached for me under the covers, I'd sighed. "Not in the mood," I'd said, desire replaced by a laser focus on my child's health. Mona's warning to prioritize our relationship went unacknowledged.

Then, one night, something newly ominous clouded the horizon. The three of us were watching television in the living room, having just finished dinner. Faith walked away. Theo and I looked at each other—our ears following the progress of her feet from the carpet onto the hard wood into her bathroom. The door shut. *Click.*

"Faith went to the bathroom," he said.

"I know," I said.

"What's she doing in there?"

"I don't know. Going to the bathroom, maybe."

I stared at the television, could feel Theo staring at me.

He kept staring at me. Aggrieved, I headed down the hallway, standing outside the door, listening to my daughter inside the bathroom like some kind of weirdo stalker. One minute went by. Another. I couldn't hear anything, like the sound of toilet paper being unfurled or pee falling into the bowl. Mona's instruction to avoid power struggles rang in my head. I knew she was right, but the living of her instruction was an altogether different matter. And, I mean, really. What magical power did Theo think I possessed, anyway? But maybe, if I could make myself sound sincere enough, I could entice her out of there without incident.

I gently tapped on the door. "You okay in there?"

"Yeah," she said.

"Need anything?"

"No. Go away."

I turned toward the living room, and that's when I heard it: the telltale sound of purposeful vomiting. Purging. My stomach clenched; my chest ached.

I returned to my spot on the couch. Faith came back. I looked at her. I'd like to believe my facial expression radiated concern. But what it probably radiated, at least to her, was judgment, anger, frustration. She glowered at me, defiant, like I was no one she wanted to know. Assumptions made in the abyss of silence. We turned back toward the TV.

We kept following Mona's protocols. "Time to go," I'd call to Faith. Regardless of where we were headed, she would scowl. I couldn't blame her. Who wants to be forced to spill their guts to strangers? Every day, she'd slam the car door. Boney Peak watched me back out of the driveway into the cul-de-sac of our self-contained, safe little neighborhood. Ten tidy houses with ten tidy lawns separated on either side by tidy green hedges. Down the tree-lined street: to and from school and swimming, to and from therapy and nutrition appointments. Getting out, she'd slam the car door. Getting in, she'd slam it again. Then back down the tree-lined street, back into the driveway. Everyone else went about their lives. We went to appointments.

Maybe it was a month or six weeks after Faith started seeing Mona, maybe longer. What I know for sure is that Faith ate a lot of crackers. Disgusted, she screamed, "I HATE MYSELF! I DON'T DESERVE TO BE ALIVE." Then she punched herself in the stomach, ran to the bathroom. I followed, but not fast enough. She'd locked the door.

"Faith," I said to the barrier of wood, "of course you deserve to be alive."

She was crying. I knocked. She ignored me. I waited and waited. She stopped crying, and I heard her sit on the floor. I sat on the floor too. Leaned my shoulder and my head against the closed door.

Minutes passed. More minutes passed. My butt throbbed. The door felt cool against my cheek. The doorjamb, I noticed, was full of divots, nicks, and chips. Beyond, the hallway closet door stuck. In the spare room, the blinds were broken.

"Sweetheart," I begged. "Please let me in."

"No," she whimpered, her voice level with my ear.

I imagined her, my mirror image: alone, scared, hurting, confused, angry. I heard her shift positions, heard the rush of my blood reverberating against the wood.

"Babe, I want to help you."

"You can't."

My sorrow was unbearable. I needed something to hate, craved hitting, ripping, attacking, punching, kicking, screaming. Needed something to *do*. I hated the fucking door, wanted to smash the bathroom to bits. I hated scales (ours, now hidden at Mona's direction in the garage), mirrors, and toilets. My inability to coax her out enraged me—the girly, light pink paint I'd chosen with toddler Faith in mind now obscene. From the wall, Winnie the Pooh was mocking me.

I dreaded the upcoming holidays; knew there'd be no special meals, no pumpkin pie or eggnog. For the first time, no presents under the tree from Mom. There'd just be more days like this one.

BATTLE ARMOR

Every soldier needs a kit. Mine was leather: big, black, Coach. A gift from a former boss. Before Faith's diagnosis, for years and years, I'd run out the door, purse in hand, willy-nilly. I always had my wallet and the tchotchkes Faith had made for me in preschool: plastic beads of purple, pink, blue, and orange strung on plastic string. If I was lucky, maybe a pen. What an ill-prepared person I'd been, running out the door that way, taking everything for granted.

After Mom died, in her purse I found a small photo keeper. Black leather with a red heart in the middle. I opened it. On the left, in a heart-shaped window, a picture I recognized of her and Bob. I'd taken it during that trip to Hawaii—of red outfit fame. They were standing in front of lush foliage, wearing shell leis. Mom's giant smile, all tooth, reminded me of when she'd admitted that she never smiled for pictures in a way that revealed her teeth because they were crooked and she was embarrassed. Faith was a baby when she'd told me that, and I'd never noticed her culled photo-smile until she pointed it out. I felt sad for her then, imagining Mom pursing her lips every time someone grabbed a camera. The insecurity. The restraint. Where had that reaction come from?

But standing over her purse, seeing that big, beautiful smile after she died made me wonder about what had changed and when. And, of course, why. Made me wonder about noticing. Or not noticing. Or only noticing in retrospect. I told Bob I was taking the photo keeper, and I transferred the memories Mom had been collecting from her purse to mine.

Now, after her death and after Faith's diagnosis, I could cry at the drop of a hat, never had a tissue when I needed one. I could no longer afford the cockiness of life from before. I dumped the contents of my big, black Coach bag onto the living room floor. There wasn't much to sort, but I threw away the lint, an errant receipt, and an empty mint wrapper. I replaced my wallet, the tchotchkes, the pen, and the compact. Added a huge wad of tissues. Oh. And always at the ready: a book.

Current selection: *Eating with Your Anorexic*, by Laura Collins.

1972

Mom said I was old enough to follow her number one rule: Stay in our yard. She didn't feel well, so she sent me outside to play. Dad was living at the scary place in New York.

I was four years old, and my puffy coat went *squee squee squee* as I walked around kicking brown, red, and yellow leaves. Next to our lake, I dug in the grass for small rocks. I missed Dad so much my chest hurt. I cried myself to sleep a lot, and whenever I told Mom I wanted Dad to come home she shrugged. I didn't like that. At night, I'd be crying and she'd tell me to stop. She'd say stuff about doing her best and about me being fine and about why couldn't I understand. I didn't like that either. I wasn't fine, and I didn't know what she meant about doing her best. I only knew that, except for Bumpy, without Dad, I felt alone.

I stood at the lake's edge, looking out. It wasn't a big lake; I could see the other side. The water was dark brown; leafy green pads and flowers floated in the middle. Ducks. Geese. And my favorites: a pair of swans. Mom and Dad said the water wasn't clean enough to swim in. That was okay. There were other lakes nearby for swimming and it was too cold now, anyway. I could see bugs land on the surface and fly away.

I threw a rock, watched the ripples spreading out. I loved how the sun sparkled on the water. The next rock I tried to skip, but without Dad's help it just sank. Dad was good at everything, including skipping rocks. Without him, I was bored. I wished I could fish, but I wouldn't put the worm on the hook. Mom always did that part for me. I went exploring by neighbor Pete's. That's when I saw something under the pricker bush and climbed in to get it.

"Tracey," Mom called from the house. "Time to come in."

I turned to obey her. I wanted to please my mom, for her to be happy with me. Maybe then, Daddy could come home.

My coat snagged on the prickers. I couldn't move.

"I'm stuck!"

I tried to move again, felt the prickers dig deeper into my jacket—prick, prick. I heard them poking holes through the fabric.

Mom called out again: "Tracey. Let's go."

She must not have heard me. "Mom, I need help!" I yelled louder.

I was afraid the prickers would rip my coat and scratch me. If my coat ripped, I'd get in trouble. If I got scratched, it would hurt. I might bleed. But Mom sounded angry. Why wasn't she paying attention? My stomach ached. Tears ran down my face.

"Get in here now!" she hollered.

But all I could do was stand there, crying, trapped and waiting to be rescued.

Finally, Mom was coming my way. Her face didn't look mean, but it didn't look nice either. I must have done something wrong. She parted the branches and helped to free me.

In silence, we walked back to the house.

WARMING

It was late and I was in bed, reading. Theo had fallen asleep on the couch. Faith walked in, stood at the threshold. Pajamas. Makeup free. She looked younger than her age, more vulnerable.

"Hi, sweetheart," I said. "You okay?"

"Can I sleep with you tonight?" she asked.

"Absolutely." A wave of tenderness washed over me. I put my book down.

Faith snuggled under the comforter, in Theo's spot, like she used to when she was little. For years, we'd struggled with baby and toddler Faith's sleep routine. At bedtime, every night, just as I was about to turn off the light, she'd strike up her little-self version of a conversation, or cry. Night after night after night, I'd walked in circles around the house, Faith in my arms, whispering and patting and bouncing until I thought my legs might cave. Once, desperate, for all of about ten minutes, I'd attempted the Ferber method: abandoning Faith to cry it out. *Oh, hell no.*

We took to the car, driving around in circles for an hour, sometimes longer. But many, many nights, Theo, returning home from work, seeing me yawn, would tell me to take her to our bed. There, I counted piggies, raspberried her belly, and kissed her palms, like Chester's mom does in a book given to us by my mom, *The Kissing Hand*. Faith would babble, shriek, and laugh until eventually we drifted off to sleep while Theo, without animus, slept on the couch.

Now, Faith wiggled closer to me, rested her cheek on my shoulder. "I have to take care of you and Dad," she blurted out. This close up, I could see how sad she looked, how tired. These days, she was always tired. And cold.

"No," I replied definitively. I wasn't sure where this was coming from. Perhaps it was because Theo and I had been butting heads more often since the drama queen comment. "It may not seem like it right now, but Dad and I will take care of each other, and we will take care of you too. That's our job. You don't need to worry about us."

"I feel so guilty. This is all my fault."

"Absolutely not," I said, the ceiling fan whirring above us. "Did you wake up one day and say to yourself, 'I'm going to give myself an eating disorder'?"

She shook her head.

"Exactly. There's nothing you need to worry about except getting better. We'll take care of the rest."

She laced her cold fingers between my cool ones. Maybe I was doing something right after all. We were quiet then, and I concentrated on the smell of eucalyptus Noxzema and mint toothpaste. On our hands, together, warming.

ALWAYS, MONEY

Thanksgiving came and went. No fanfare. No special food. No communion with family. Then it was December. Faith went to school but came home and disintegrated into tears, yelling, or jumping jacks. Or all three. After swim, she said it wasn't hard enough or that she was too slow or that everyone else was better than she was. Everyone was better at everything than she was.

Everyone was skinnier. Everyone was smarter and more talented. Everyone had a boyfriend. She was the only girl in her entire school who was "ugly and alone." Her joints sometimes made weird popping noises that I attributed to the overexercising and inconsistent nutrition. She started encircling her left wrist with her right thumb and middle finger as a way to gauge her size—the more the thumb could overlap the middle fingernail, the better. I found a drawing she made on her bedroom floor, a self-portrait, except she'd drawn herself in the shape of the Pillsbury Doughboy. But there was only one doughboy in this family.

We kept driving, kept going to appointments. Southern California. No foul, freezing weather to slow us down. Out of the driveway, down the tree-lined street, and onto the 101 Freeway. On our left, the mall. On our right, the golf course. I kept waiting, in the waiting room or in the car. And I continued to see my therapist, Kim, keeping her abreast of developments. To her, I cried. She was the only person I felt safe enough with to fully express my emotions. Even though I knew the answer, I wondered why treatment was taking so long, when things would change for the better, and what it would take for Faith to improve. The answer being: it would take as long as it took.

At the end of every session, she'd remind me that Faith wanted to see me taking care of myself. If she tired of saying the same thing, it never showed on her face. When no one else was home, instead of taking care of myself, I'd grab cookies from the pantry, slices of cheese from the fridge, ice cream from the freezer, or peanut M&M's from Theo's secret stash, making up for what lacked at mealtimes.

Mona's pronouncement, toward the middle of December, didn't surprise me. It scared me. "The plan isn't working," she said. She'd called me to this meeting to tell me we had to try something else. Theo was working a freelance gig, and as much as I didn't want to hear those words, I knew she was right. Mona handed me a brochure for a residential treatment center in Arizona.

"Nope," I said.

I still thought residential treatment was too severe a step. I wouldn't consider sending my daughter, an eighth grader, away from our home, let alone out of the state. After discussing the available options in our community, we settled on an outpatient eating disorder clinic called the LV Center.

At home, I filled Theo in. "She's forcing our hand," he said, rubbing his head—a nervous habit. He meant that Faith's behaviors were requiring stronger interventions, and he was right; although, scary as it was, I preferred to think about it as the illness taking more control—a subtle but important distinction. We discussed the idea of residential treatment and came to one conclusion: we couldn't imagine what would change our mind about something as serious as that.

I called the LV Center for an appointment to enroll Faith in the intensive program—five days a week after school and Saturday mornings—thinking again that *this* would be the fix we needed. Over the phone, LV's intake coordinator took our insurance information and said they'd call back with an appointment time only after our benefit level was confirmed. I envisioned the person on the other end of the line, hitting the mute button to yell, "Show me the money!"

Money. First. Last. Always. What recourse would we have, I wondered, but for adequate resources?

PART TWO

SHEER FORCE OF WILL

Despite our better judgment, I had accepted an invitation for the three of us. New Year's Eve, a friend's surprise birthday dinner, a restaurant Faith had always loved with a singing waitstaff. "Yes, please," Theo and I had said to each other, to our friends.

We'd wanted to spend a few hours being ordinary, doing an ordinary thing. And we'd felt certain that a break would also benefit Faith. Obviously, of late not much had been fun.

The transition from Mona to the LV Center had caused more upset, more tears, more upheaval, and without the structure of school during winter vacation, disruption was layered on top of disruption. For the dinner out, we had prepared, of course. For everyone attending LV, the year-end conversations in group and family therapy sessions had centered almost exclusively on the holidays, food, and planning. The preparations had ameliorated some of Faith's anxiety. She hadn't exactly had fun at the restaurant, but neither had she seemed miserable. And she hadn't overeaten. Home from the early dinner in time to watch the ball drop, Theo and I fell asleep thinking we'd be okay.

But now, in the harsh light of day, Faith was stalking the house—from her room to the backyard to the living room, and back again. When not stalking, she slumped on the couch, her head hanging, staring at nothing.

"My stomach is sticking out so far," she moaned.

It wasn't, but I kept my mouth shut.

"I hate myself," she said. "Why can't I be normal, like everyone else?"

"Wanna watch Food Network?" Theo asked.

"No," she growled.

"Why don't you write in your journal?" I asked.

"Fuck no," she said.

"Watch your language," Theo said.

Foul language was a symptom of Faith's depression, and Mona had suggested we institute consequences for disrespectful behavior. But I'd disagreed on the grounds of hypocrisy. Faith had grown up hearing Theo and I sometimes swear, and comparatively speaking, bad words seemed like the least of our problems. She said using profanity made her feel better. It always made me feel better too.

"Want to play a game?" I offered.

"Stop talking," she said.

"Let's play guitar," Theo said.

"Take a shower?" I asked, reaching out to touch her.

"Don't touch me!" she yelled.

She jumped up to resume pacing.

This dance—Faith struggling to keep herself in check while Theo and I watched, waited—went on for hours, the house a pressure cooker. We suggested every available tool at our disposal. Nothing penetrated the barrier of the illness.

Faith dropped down in front of the couch, gave an earth-shattering shriek. She punched the pillows with all her might. I rushed to her, murmuring words of encouragement. Theo snapped to attention.

Faith rocked back onto her heels, an odd calm washing over her features. I wasn't sure if she recognized me. She stood, heading for the hallway. A chill ran down my spine. I followed.

She stepped into her bathroom, tried to close the door, but I blocked it.

She kept pushing. "Leave . . . me . . . alone," she grunted.

"Not gonna happen." I gritted my teeth. Whatever she planned to do in there couldn't be good. I was going to win this one, no matter what.

She let go of the door, looked at herself in the mirror. "I can see myself getting fatter. Oh, god," she cried. "I can't go on like this. What's wrong with me? There's something wrong with me, Mom. You have to do something. You have to help me kill myself." She punched herself in the stomach.

I launched myself into the bathroom, but she was too quick. She bashed her head into the tile wall, wobbled backward.

I shouted to Theo, "Make the call!"

Both Mona and the new clinicians at the LV Center had told Theo and me to call 911 if we felt that Faith was becoming unsafe toward herself or us. *Like hell I will.* I'd refused to admit to myself that we wouldn't be able to help her. But now . . .

I heard Theo yell on the phone, "It's my daughter!"

Faith collapsed into a heap on the floor, crying. I sat on the toilet, crying.

She rested her head in my lap. I stroked the lump on her forehead—the first time all day she'd accepted my touch. Later, she would tell me she was trying to knock the bad thoughts out. But now, we waited to find out what would happen next.

The doorbell rang. *Clomp-clomp.* Work boots heading toward us.

A paramedic's reflective jacket stepped into my sight line. *Woman?! Good.* Perhaps Faith would be more comfortable talking to a woman. The paramedic kneeled down in front of us, set a machine on the floor. Her trained eyes assessed the scene. She made that weird *cluck-tsk* sound people make when they feel bad but know words won't help.

"Are you hurt anywhere?" she asked Faith.

"I have a headache."

In the background, I heard Theo explaining that he'd called because of our daughter's depression and eating disorder. "We're doing everything we can, but it's not working," he said, an imploring quality to his voice I'd never heard.

The woman shined a small light in Faith's eyes, then took her blood pressure, pulse rate, and temperature. Finally, she performed a head and neck exam. I remained on the toilet, my hand on Faith's back, until another medic called me into the hallway.

He asked me for details Theo had already given: Faith's name, age, school. Was this guy assessing me? *Does he think* I *hurt her? That I was drunk? Hungover?* It was New Year's Day, after all.

I was clearheaded as could be. Theo was still sober, and as Faith had gotten sicker, I'd sworn off alcohol too. I needed to be alert. The guy was just doing his job, but still.

Meanwhile, the woman paramedic said, "Do you have a plan to kill yourself?"

She was talking to my daughter.

"No," Faith whimpered. Barely audible: "I just wish I wasn't here."

My muscles, bones, and blood panicked.

"Have you cut yourself?" the woman asked her.

"Yes."

"Can I see?"

Faith pulled up her left sleeve. My eyes widened; my hand flew to my mouth. From elbow to wrist, her forearm was scratched and red, as if she'd played a fiendish game of tic-tac-toe on her flesh. She'd done this to herself—I'd had no idea. At this first glimpse of the injuries, I fell into the trap I could usually avoid. *How could she?*

Physically, Faith was fine. She hadn't given herself a concussion. The scratches were superficial. The paramedics packed up their gear, wished us well. I imagined they were thinking, *There are real problems in the world, car wrecks and gunshot wounds.* My face flushed with shame and embarrassment. Two policemen had arrived shortly after the paramedics. One of them suggested Faith should probably get evaluated at the county hospital, thirty miles away. Theo and I looked at each other. We had nothing more to go on than instinct, but where instinct ended and fear began, who knew. After a debate lasting twenty minutes and our promise not to take our eyes off of our daughter, they departed.

Faith crawled into our bed, fell instantly asleep. I crawled in next to her. Staring up, I watched the ceiling fan rotate, noticed that 1970s-era popcorn soundproofing. I listened to her breathe. In and out. Slow and steady. Tears dripped down my temples onto my pillow. Everything, as my dad used to say, was going to hell in a handbasket.

The image of Faith's scratches skittered across my mind, and the stabbing pain under my right shoulder hurt worse than ever. I remembered seeing that one long scratch, the previous year, on her wrist. Would anything be different now if I'd done something or said something else then? Why hadn't I? There were no guarantees, but my decision felt like another mistake in a growing string of mistakes.

I blotted my eyes with my sleeve, gently rolled onto my side. Undisturbed, Faith slumbered on—at peace, finally. In the dim light of the night-light, my eyes traced her profile: forehead, nose (Theo's), mouth (mine), chin. Why? Why was this happening? When would this nightmare end? *Please.*

Whom was I begging? Not God. I'd long since relinquished my connection to the Catholicism of my childhood. Mom? Dad? Faith said she didn't want to be here. I was trying to protect my daughter, but was I? I wasn't so sure. *What am I supposed to do?*

There seemed to be only one answer: keep her alive, by myself if necessary, with the sheer force of my will.

MORE

The next day, I called the LV Center to tell Faith's newest therapist about the 911 call and the scratches. She assured me she'd alert the rest of the team and instructed me to collect and hide anything sharp from Faith's bedroom and bathroom.

Dutifully, Theo and I scoured drawers, cabinets, and cubbyholes for razors, nail clippers, scissors, tweezers, thumbtacks, paper clips, staples, lapel pins, broken pieces of plastic, bits of this and that. We must have debated and decried this latest development, must have withered in the realization, kitchen aside, of exactly how many sharp objects resided inside our home. At some point, Theo looked at me and said, "Darling, she's going to be okay."

I wasn't sure what about my face or posture compelled him to say so, but I leaned into him, resting my cheek on his chest, upheld by his strength.

That day and in the days to come, we must have talked to Faith about using positive methods to cope—that's what the therapy was about. We never said out loud that we wanted her to hurry up and get better, or that we wanted the process to speed up. We knew the truth, same as before: it would take as long as it took. And yet. In gesture and tone, we must have conveyed impatience and, as hard as it is to admit, anger—our lives were in total disarray. But we did agree out loud, to each other and to Faith, if she needed something, like a razor to shave, she would have to ask and we'd watch her use it.

Faith returned to school after winter break—depression running roughshod over daily life. Her head hung. She never smiled, and began forgetting basic hygiene practices. And she never sang. She had, as I'd hoped, memorized *The Book of Mormon* soundtrack. Gloriously, several times during that process, her clear alto had wafted down the hallway. But in the two months since then, not one note. She rarely spoke at all, really, except to say that she hated Mona for suggesting the LV Center. She hated us for making her go. She hated the therapists there. The girls there hated her. But most of all, she hated herself. Hearing Faith berate herself broke my heart. I tried not to argue with her; arguing invalidated her feelings. I usually failed, unable to tolerate the pain her pain was causing me.

The LV Center was located on the ground floor of a nondescript two-story office building in the town adjacent to ours. Aside from the steady stream of young girls walking in and out, nothing indicated an eating disorder clinic.

The program required more. More therapy. In addition to individual therapy, Faith was required to join daily group sessions, and Theo and I were required to attend weekly couples therapy, and for the three of us, together, weekly family therapy and weekly family group sessions with the other clinic clients. More participation. If we seemed reluctant to speak, we were called on. More suspicion. Theo and I were interviewed, together and apart, about Faith's history, whether abuse of any kind existed. As far as we knew, none did, which didn't stop us from feeling like criminals, looking at one other and other people like criminals, and combing memories of our past for potential clues, disturbed to have another terrifying concern planted in our minds.

I realized that we were not the only family dealing with a

child's mental health condition. This fact should have ameliorated my feelings of shame, inadequacy, and responsibility. But it didn't. Also at this time, as part of LV's program, a psychiatrist prescribed Faith an antidepressant. As reluctant as we were, Theo and I signed off.

The new routine: Every day after school, I'd drop Faith off at LV, go home and make dinner. The program didn't provide food, so I would separate out Faith's portion, sling my purse over my shoulder, and drive back to deliver the food piping hot and fresh. While Faith ate with the other girls and therapists, so they could work together through eating issues and emotions, I would return home to eat with Theo. We'd sit in front of the TV, too drained usually for idle chitchat.

But when we spoke, we often argued. We argued about how to handle ourselves in reaction to Faith's behaviors, the extent to which those behaviors were related to her illness, and about her ability to control them—no closer to being in the same book, let alone on the same page. At the end of the day, finally, Theo or I would pick Faith up and bring her home, where she'd go to her room and slam the door.

Mondays were spaghetti and homemade turkey meatballs day. We stuck to a rigid menu plan so Faith would always know what she'd be eating. One or two Mondays after the New Year's Day 911 call, I dumped a container of ground turkey into a mixing bowl. I cracked in an egg, added a sprinkle of breadcrumbs and pinches of fresh-ground salt and pepper and Italian seasoning. I smelled the earthy oregano.

Before the LV Center, Faith would watch me prepare dinner to ensure that I didn't sneak anything fattening in—not the modus operandi prior to her diagnosis. But now I grabbed the container of grated parmesan cheese, tossed in a couple of tablespoons. The pediatrician and the nutritionist had explained to Faith that fat is a necessary component of a healthy diet, and I did try to sneak some in. People at LV were monitoring Faith's weight, which still appeared unchanged. A sprinkle of cheese wouldn't change much, except for making me feel better.

Plunging my hands into the gooey concoction, I folded everything together. Food. Buying it. Preparing it. Eating it. Enjoying it. Despising it. My weight hadn't stopped me from achieving life's major milestones like graduating from high school and college with honors, obtaining good jobs, getting married, and having a healthy baby. But it had underpinned decisions I'd made regarding everything from what to wear and how to act, to where to go and who to like.

Doing internet research, I'd stumbled upon the National Association of Anorexia Nervosa and Associated Disorders website, a statistic: twenty-four million people in the course of their lifetime would have an eating disorder. A number so huge it was incomprehensible. Were there millions of moms out there right now, daughters and sons too, going through what we were?

I spread a couple of baking sheets out on the counter, started rolling raw meat into one-inch balls. Another and another. The rhythm soothed me, and, lost in thought, I remembered the tiny kitchen of my childhood home. It was a fraction of the size of mine, the one Theo had enlarged and remodeled, by himself, as my wedding gift. I had no idea how Mom had prepared meals in there. It was barely big enough for the appliances and a small table, avocado green as I recalled.

I didn't remember my mother as someone who had enjoyed cooking when I was a kid, maybe because I'd rarely enjoyed what she made. A few things I'd liked: her special-recipe meatloaf, lentil soup with cut-up hot dogs, and holiday apple pie with handmade dough and extra cinnamon. But I'd hated her stinky baked fish and disgusting canned Veg-All. "Blech," I would say, out loud. To which she'd frown. "I went out of my way to make that. You could show some appreciation." I'd squirm, feeling guilty, roll peas around my plate. Hold my nose, swallow.

It was the 1970s. Mom must have been in that kitchen every day, but, as with most things related to my childhood, it was Dad who stood out. Even there. His salt-and-pepper-colored hair gleaming in the overhead light. Sunday morning silver dollar–size pancakes. Butter. Jelly. Whistling. He whistled while he shined his shoes, played piano, cooked—a skill, he'd often said, honed during his years as a tank commander in World War II.

I would listen, watch, eat. Pop those bite-size goodnesses into my mouth whole, one after the other, never get full, and listen to my parents argue, often about me and food. I'd never been able to decide what made me feel worse: being the thorn in their relationship or being overweight.

Back in my own kitchen, neat rows of bite-size meatballs lined both cookie sheets. I popped them into the oven, checked the clock. I had plenty of time left to complete the meal and deliver it to Faith. I looked forward to returning home, heaping my plate with spaghetti, lots of sauce, and several meatballs. I'd pair it with a big bowl of salad, sprinkle everything with another healthy dose of parmesan. Then more, with seconds. I knew I was using food to distract myself, to numb. But there was more to the cycle than that.

My first therapist, Dolly, and I had unpacked my cyclical relationship with food: feel bad—eat—feel bad—eat. We looked into the past, and for the first time I was able to acknowledge and articulate my ruminations about food, my body, and my parents. I was thirty-one years old when Dolly suggested there were reasons I used food the way that I did, which were not, as I had suspected, because I was a lazy person who just liked to eat a lot. I wasn't sure I believed her, had felt guilty just talking about my childhood. What did I have to complain about? I'd had a roof over my head, food on the table—everything a kid could ask for.

But Dolly had taught me we find comfort in what we're used to, and, after decades of practice, I was comfortable obsessing about dieting rather than feeling like a shitty, inadequate person and mother.

Ten years after Dolly, this habituated pattern took over, again. Crisis changes the way our brain functions. Deep-seated instincts for self-preservation kick in. It was never my conscious intent to crawl into bed and ruminate, as I tried to fall asleep, about how full and how fat I was rather than how afraid I felt, but that's exactly what would happen.

BATTLE ARMOR, KIT ADDITIONS

Checkbook
Small notepad
Current selection: *Beautiful Boy*, by David Sheff

1980

Stupid Dr. Emma and her stupid diet.

I was sick of turkey sandwiches, baked chicken breast, broiled fish, and cottage cheese. I stood at the threshold to the kitchen and looked in at the refrigerator, the cabinets, the stove. I wanted to stay away, to make Mom and Dad proud of me. But when it came to the kitchen, I was a moth to the flame: pumpernickel bread, Nutter Butter cookies, candy cigarettes. Mom could hardly complain about those, considering what a smoke stack she was.

You're gross, I said to myself. And, *Don't be a pig*. And, *Stay away from the cookies. Eat an apple!* I was trying to get myself to listen, and I didn't understand why it wasn't working.

At the table, my parents would speak of me as if I were not even there.

"Jerry," Mom would say, casting a concerned look in my direction, saying that "we" had better be careful.

"Lauraine," Dad would say.

You tell her, Dad, I'd think. At least he loved me the way I was. Why couldn't she? The difference was confusing.

"That's not on your diet," Mom would say, and "Are you sure you want that?" and "Don't you want to look like your friends?" Of course I wanted to look like my friends, and the beautiful skinny actresses on TV. But if I complained, she'd tell me to stop being so sensitive. I gave up.

"Look," Dad said one time to Mom. "She's just built like my side of the family, a brick shithouse."

I scanned his face for signs of disappointment. But I didn't see any. I thought maybe "brick shithouse" wasn't too bad. Maybe he was trying to make Mom be quiet, like, *Don't talk that way about my daughter!* I could almost always count on him to make me feel better, to make me laugh. Or maybe he was trying to make Mom feel better by saying I wasn't her fault. Either way, Mom looked annoyed.

She pushed her chair back. "She'd be so pretty if she lost weight."

WHAC-A-MOLE

I was picking Faith's pajamas up off the floor—tidiness, like good personal hygiene, no longer interested her—when I saw it. We were still just a couple of weeks into the New Year, and I had dropped her off at school. Something on the sweatshirt material had caught my eye.

I took a closer look: a half-dollar-size spot of blood on one of the sleeves. Flummoxed, I rubbed my thumb across it. I held the shirt up. More spots of blood. Realization shrouded my brain like a wet wool blanket.

I whipped around, searching for the culprit, for what she'd used to hurt herself. Found nothing. *Fix this*, my inner voice commanded.

Like an automaton, I gathered a dark laundry load, carried it to the garage, and stuffed everything but the shirt into the washing machine. I smeared generous globs of Stain Stick onto the bloody spots. Massaged the goo into the fabric's fibers. A light scent of iron reached my nostrils, turning my stomach. I dropped the shirt into the washer, set the dial, and washed my hands in the kitchen sink.

Back in Faith's room, I was about to make the bed when I saw droplets of dried blood on the sheet. I ripped off the sheets and pillowcases, walked back to the garage. Standing at the machine, I bit my lip and furiously rubbed more Stain Stick into the cotton fibers. Inside my body, a feeling seemed to emanate from my cells. *Tick. Tick. Tick.* An imaginary stopwatch was counting down the seconds. I was racing against time, running a marathon without instruction or training. What might meet me beyond the finish line? I couldn't bear to contemplate. But I could do laundry.

The washing machine and dryer worked all morning.

I called the director of the LV Center to alert her about my discovery. "It's normal," she said.

"Normal?" I said.

"Self-harming behavior escalates as disordered eating behavior de-escalates. It's a game of Whac-A-Mole. One behavior goes down and a different one pops up."

"Good analogy," I said, with a dark chuckle. It was either that or let loose about the actual meaning of normal.

Later, I filled Theo in. "This is so fucked up," he said.

"Yes," I said. "It is."

YESTERDAY, TODAY, TOMORROW

"You're sure doing a lot of laundry," Theo said. "Didn't you just do a load?"

THE BOTTOM

I considered buying one of those cop show devices—the snake camera that can slide under doors. But before it came to that, LV's director called us into a meeting to say that Faith had to be pulled out of school.

"She needs intensive outpatient treatment—to be here all day, not just the afternoons," Holly said.

I recoiled. "What about her education?"

"An education won't matter if she kills herself," Holly said.

BATTLE ARMOR, KIT ADDITIONS

Band-Aids
ChapStick
Cough drops

INVISIBLE TO VISIBLE

Amy, our family therapist at the LV Center, sat across from Theo, Faith, and me. The realization that Faith was now hurting herself enough to draw blood, with what object we didn't know and hadn't been able to find, had changed everything. And nothing.

What else could we do? She was now attending treatment five days a week all day and Saturday mornings. Theo and I attended every week's couples, family, and family group sessions. They'd advised us to always leave Faith's bedroom door open, and we'd threatened to follow through on removing it entirely. The bathroom door could be closed enough to shield view of the toilet but needed to be left ajar. Every time she was in her room, like a palace guardsman, I paraded back and forth in front of the opening every ten minutes or so.

"Why do you think she's cutting?" Amy asked.

"To hurt us," Theo replied.

I clenched my teeth, butted in. "I don't think that's it. I think she's trying to take all that pain that's in her head and make it real on her body."

Amy nodded. "This is a real way for her to show you how much pain she's actually in."

She's not the only one, I thought, as Amy explained that self-harm was a messed-up way to cope. Faith sighed, rolled her eyes. Her legs jackhammered up and down with anxiety. Amy went on to say that cutting, as strange as it sounded, helped people deal with intense, overwhelming emotions and was addictive in the sense that over time people needed more to achieve the calming result. If anyone on the treatment team at this point was openly comparing self-harm's addictive nature to Theo's alcoholism and mine with food and ruminating, I don't remember them doing so. Even if they had, the likelihood is I would have missed the point, as distracted as I was.

Amy went on to say that generally speaking, the behavior was not considered a suicide attempt, but it had to be taken very seriously. Statements like that—*Self-harm has to be taken seriously*—and other pithy quips like, *Feelings aren't facts*, bugged the absolute shit out of me. Of course we were taking the situation seriously. We could not take it any more seriously. Our child had said she wished she wasn't alive. Whenever Amy questioned Faith now in family sessions about suicidality or having a plan to end her life, Faith responded the same way, "I don't have a plan, but I wish I'd never been born." Theo and I sat there, stone-faced, while our hearts shattered.

This particular session ended with the adults reminding Faith to use the healthy tools she was learning—therapy and art and writing and music—to cope rather than cutting herself. Faith agreed, though we figured she was telling us what we wanted to hear.

1978

Instead of going to my pediatrician, this time Mom took me to the emergency room. Dr. Emma never could figure out why my stomach hurt, why I sometimes threw up. She'd ruled out food poisoning a long time ago because it happened too often for that, and Mom and Dad never got sick. But I must have been crying and complaining a lot to end up in the hospital.

Mom held my hand because I was scared. She said not to be afraid, the doctors would help me like they'd helped Dad after his heart attack. Seeing him in the hospital, finally, after I'd begged, I found him pale and weak, almost as white as the sheet, with tubes in his arms. I was terrified, but also comforted when he reached his hand to touch my face. He was home now, getting stronger every day.

I was on the exam bed, Mom standing next to me, still holding my hand. It was bright in there, so bright my eyes almost hurt. And cold. I shivered under the light blanket, but I didn't complain. The whole place stunk like chemicals, and I wanted to go home.

I wanted to believe Mom about the doctor helping me, but I was afraid that if something was wrong with me, she'd leave me there. I remembered getting my tonsils out. The awful mask they put over my face. I was crying, and they did it anyway. I tried to hold my breath because the gas smelled so bad. They told me to count backward from one hundred, but I floated away when I got to ninety-seven. When I woke up, my throat was killing me. I felt woozy and sick. Threw up. Actually, I felt a lot like that now. Woozy. Nauseous. Why couldn't anyone tell me why my stomach hurt?

A nurse came, took my temperature, left. Next, a doctor. He had a clipboard and a pen. He told my mom I didn't have a fever, but we knew that already. I never had a fever when I felt like this. He asked her questions and then he asked me more questions. He pushed around on my stomach, said everything seemed fine. Then he asked me, "Does your bottom hurt or itch when you go to the bathroom? Could be a tapeworm."

My eyes got big. A worm? Inside me? *No, no, no.* That could not be true. I looked at Mom. She smiled reassuringly. I looked up at the ceiling. My face felt hot. Sometimes it did itch, but I wasn't going to admit that to this guy. Even if he was a doctor. "No," I said.

He said I seemed fine in a tone that suggested I might be telling tales. He probably told Mom to make sure I drank a lot of water. She probably gave him her *I can only do my best* face. She was still holding my hand when we stepped into the hallway. I had enough time to say, "Uh-oh."

I barfed. Twice. Goo spread across the hallway. I started crying. Bits got on my shoes. "I'm sorry," I cried. *See?*

A nurse came with a couple of paper towels, smiled at me. She seemed nice, and I thought, *That won't be enough paper towels for this mess.*

SEARCHING

The search continued: drawers, bookshelves, boxes, bags, purses, jewelry box, medicine chest. Ideally, the therapists said, Faith would choose to surrender the object or objects she was using. A week went by, maybe two, so this was late January, and surrendering seemed less and less likely; I kept finding evidence on clothes, sheets, towels, tissues, and Band-Aids.

In addition to removing the obvious sharp objects like razors and pushpins, leaving doors open, and possibly removing them completely, we were told to ignore the behavior. That anyone could expect parents to ignore potentially life-threatening behavior is ludicrous, but my brain says it's true. More likely, the actual conversation swirled around control, as it had since the very beginning. We were to avoid power struggles.

But nothing about this was ideal, so Theo and I searched. When Faith was home, his anxiety erupted into a steady stream of reportage. "Faith went to the bathroom. What's she doing in there? She's been in there for a while. Can't you get her out of there?"

"Do I look like I have X-ray vision?" I'd finally snap. "*You* go ask her."

"I'm not supposed to say anything, remember?"

He'd been instructed by Mona and the therapists at LV to walk away if he couldn't stop riding me, if he couldn't stop complaining about the effects of Faith's behavior on *him*, implying that she could change if she just wanted to badly enough and if she faced her character defects and accepted she had a problem.

On Theo went: "Can't you get her out of there? You should do something. You know she's in there doing something. This is so fucked up. I am so upset."

It was hard enough for me to control myself—to not scream at Faith, to not beg her to stop. But Theo's badgering fueled the fire already burning inside me that said I had to act. Or else. That if something truly terrible transpired, it would be my fault. So I'd get off the couch, walk past Faith's bathroom and head into mine, which shared a common wall with hers, straining to figure out what she was doing. When that failed, I'd walk back to her door.

"What ya doin' in there, babe? Everything okay?"

"Yeah," she'd say. "Going to the bathroom." Or, "Leave me alone, this is my grounding space." Or, "Yep. Just, ya know, peeing."

"Okay. You've been in there for a while."

"Uh-huh."

I'd walk away, trying to balance privacy and safety.

Two more minutes.

Theo: "You've gotta get her out of there."

Sometimes I tried to be invisible. Other times I tried to be obvious. I stood vigil outside the bathroom door, willing her to make healthier choices. Or I banged on the door and pleaded for her to let me in. I stomped like a mad bull, prowled like a feral cat. These encounters resolved in one of two basic ways. Sometimes Faith really went into the bathroom to use the toilet. She'd return to the living room, and we'd resume watching whatever show was on. Hope would blossom. More often she'd head from her bathroom to mine, where we kept the first aid supplies. Hope would fizzle. Theo would threaten again to remove the doors, and I'd beg her to let me help tend the wound, which she always refused. And when she was at LV, we re-searched each nook and cranny, looking for the proverbial or real needle in a haystack.

Across from Kim, in my sweatpants and hair clip, I cried. "Why is this happening? When will it end?" Whenever Kim asked me what I could do for myself, I pointed at all the people, places, and things standing in my way. I berated Theo. "He's the adult. Faith's the kid. He should do what he's told. It feels like he's willfully ignoring instructions." I belittled the LV staff. "Who says something as stupid as, 'We have to take this seriously'? Are you fucking kidding me?" And, with an almost obsessive quality, I complained about the middle school staff.

When I'd called to withdraw Faith from eighth grade, the counselor I'd been dealing with had informed me that no other students were having the type of problem Faith was. Knowing her statement was either ignorance or a bald-faced lie made me feel no better. Every time I'd questioned the counselor about what we should be doing for my daughter's education, she'd respond the same way. "Faith's not here. There's nothing we can do."

Kim, experienced with school district policy and procedure and the law, frowned at the conclusion of one particular day's diatribe. "Here's what I want you to do," she said. "Tell her exactly this: 'My daughter's disability is preventing her from getting an education.' And let me know what happens."

I wasn't sure how I felt about that label, but it didn't matter because I trusted Kim. I would have said the moon was made out of cheese if she told me it would help Faith. Action was what I expected and action was what I got. That counselor had sighed, clearly put out, but soon enough district personnel were being contacted, meetings were being scheduled. The process for obtaining an Individualized Education Plan (IEP), which is legally binding and has a mandated timeline, to help Faith when she was ready to return to school, had begun.

But mostly, across from Kim, I searched for the solace I could not, for whatever reason, find elsewhere. I'd pull pictures of younger Faith out of my purse, practically shoving them in Kim's face. "See," I'd say. "Look how happy she looks. You can't fake a smile like that."

Sure enough, there was Faith's sweet, untroubled younger face. A giant smile. Clear blue eyes. Kim would take the picture, smile, and nod. I must have reminisced: trips to the beach, play-dates, Brownilympics. And, in an attempt to clear my conscience, I confessed.

"I saw that used Band-Aid in the trash, and I couldn't stop myself. I thought, one slap. Maybe one good hard slap might turn off the switch that turned on in Faith's brain." I hesitated, searching Kim's face for the judgment I expected to see. Seeing none, I swallowed. "That thought terrified me, but I couldn't help it. I'm a terrible person. I don't even deserve to be a mother."

"Having feelings makes you a human being," Kim said. "It's what you do or don't do with them that matters."

HELP?

Amy, during a family session: "We want you to know we're taking the cutting seriously. I've purchased a workbook with exercises for Faith to do, recording her thoughts and behaviors. It should really help."

AND EVERYTHING IN BETWEEN

Rose
Scarlet
Mahogany

Wet
Dried
Crusty

Toilet
Floor
Sink

MOM'S BIRTHDAY

"Thanks for your help," I said into the phone. I was home, sitting at my desk. "Sorry about the last-minute change."

It was early February, and I'd just canceled Faith's participation in the eighth-grade spring break field trip to Washington, D.C. I'd waited as long as possible, but there was no way she could go. She couldn't even go to school. And today should have been Mom's sixty-eighth birthday—another first without her. The losses were piling up like the bills: therapy, nutrition, doctors, LV.

My vision floated upward, to the shelf over my desk. Before Mom died, knowing how much I missed New Jersey's beautiful fall colors, she'd placed an array of red, yellow, and gold leaves on an eight-by-ten-inch piece of cardboard, covered them with clear plastic, and mailed them to me. The vibrancy had long since faded to brown, but the leaves themselves were intact. *Dear Tracey*, she'd written in cursive in the corner. *For you*.

I burst into tears, burying my face in my hands.

Theo stepped into my office, wanted to know what was wrong.

What wasn't wrong? The stupid workbook exercises hadn't made a difference, of course. Most of Faith's friends were going on the field trip, kids she wasn't seeing at all now because she was in treatment during the day instead of at school. Cancellation had such an air of finality, like we had nothing to look forward to and our situation wasn't going to improve. Mom was dead. I felt like we'd never be ordinary again. Never be able to take a vacation or even eat at a freaking restaurant, without dire consequences.

"I really wanted Faith to be able to take that trip," I said into my palms.

Theo kneeled down, put his arm around me. "Honey, you just need to be happy. Find something to be happy about."

Here we go again. I shrugged off his arm. "I told you already, don't tell me how to feel." His dedication to this inane sentiment left me cold, especially today. "Why don't *you* go find something to be happy about?"

Theo stood. He headed toward the living room. "I *am* happy. I'm on the top side of the grass." He said something about accepting my powerlessness.

"Oh, my god, don't start."

"You need a twelve-step program."

"And you need to stop talking."

I was proud of Theo's dedication to sobriety. In six years, he hadn't touched a drop of alcohol. So type A personality. So him. No matter what, Theo always followed through—the trait of his I most admired. But Theo's comment wasn't about alcohol. It was his way of telling me to be like him, to do the work he'd done—make a fearless moral inventory, admit wrongdoing, remove character defects—so that I'd be fine. Meaning: I'd be fixed. But I thought he needed to take his own advice before telling everyone else what to do. Sobriety itself hadn't improved his ability to communicate, accept what he couldn't change, or change what he could aside from alcohol consumption.

My phone rang. It was Isabelle's mom, Grace. Faith's friends had noticed her monthlong absence from school, and Grace had been reaching out. She was the only person who knew some of what was happening, but I swiped to decline. I'd dropped out of book club, had cleared my schedule. I only left the house for therapy appointments and necessary errands. I headed toward the kitchen, thinking about the happy birthday phone call I didn't need to make to Mom and the one—or was it two? More?—I'd shamefully made late. "Oh, you remembered," Mom would say, thus confirming my shitty-daughter-ness. Theo followed me, prattling on about life's unmanageability.

I yanked a few tissues from the box. "Stop!"

Theo snorted, glared at me, and stormed to the garage.

My coffee mug, its contents gone cold, sat on the counter where I'd left it hours ago. It had come to me from Mom's house after she died, and I'd been rinsing and reusing it almost daily. I was overcome with an urge to call her. After a lifetime of keeping my mother at an emotional distance, I wanted to talk to her now more than ever. It was a fantasy—expecting her to somehow be able to say what she'd never before said. After Dad died, she hadn't even said, "I'm sorry," the way folks do when someone you love dies. Most who mean it, some who don't. Regardless. I was hysterical in the aftermath. Two words from her would have acknowledged she saw my pain. That I mattered. Instead, I'd felt like I was talking to a robot.

Still, I imagined. I imagined myself picking up the phone, dialing her number. I imagined hearing her say hello. "Mom?" I'd simply have to say. "I'm on my way," she would say. I imagined not needing, even, to ask.

I imagined my mother doing what the therapists had been encouraging me to do with Faith: validate me—such a sterile word for what I craved, what I needed and had never received from my mother. Mom saying something like, "I'm always here for you. You're doing your best and that's enough. You're amazing. Faith's amazing. You two will be okay." Whether it was true or false was not the point. I wanted to hear the belief in her voice. The confidence.

I wanted to know that no matter what, my mother had my back.

APRIL 1, 1980

Dani, Gwen, and I were waiting outside school for the bell to ring. It was a beautiful spring day; leaves fluttered in the breeze. I was a few months into my diet, but I pretty much looked the same as before.

I noticed Arnie, Simon, and Dale—popular boys—standing nearby, whispering and looking our way. They had never paid us any mind. We had lots of friends, but we weren't in the popular group. I'd had a secret crush on Arnie for six years, since kindergarten. When he smiled his brown eyes got bright, mischievous. We were good friends, kidded around together in class. I let him borrow my books, and when he wouldn't give them back, we'd wrestle. I kept hoping that one day he'd like me too.

The guys headed our way. Gwen and I exchanged a confused glance. They formed a line in front of us. Arnie stood across from me. In unison they said, "Will you go out with me?"

For a second, my breath caught. Was it finally my turn?

But then the boys started laughing. "April Fools'!" they yelled, and took off running around like idiots.

We girls just shrugged, like, *Ha-ha, jerks, real funny*—pretended we didn't care. I looked around to see who was watching. A few of the other guys were sniggering. It was then that I realized what all the fuss about my body was, why Mom kept talking about fruit and why Dr. Emma looked so concerned. No popular boy would ever love a girl who looked like me. Arnie would never be mine.

Later, I made the mistake of telling Mom what had happened. I wanted her to tell me it wasn't my fault, that I was perfect the way I was. "Boys will be boys," she said. "You need to learn how to take a joke."

CERTAIN CIRCUMSTANCES

I've tried to remember more of the useful words we spoke during those early therapy sessions where Theo, Faith, and I were present. We put energy, time, and care into showing up to say them. Day after day. Week after week. We agonized over those words. What they stated outright. What they implied. What they would or would not be able to do for us and why. My journals no doubt contain clues, and with dedicated time and attention I could probably reconstruct at least some of those exchanges. But as any student of story knows: it's the image that lingers.

And the single clearest image retained in my mind from Faith's time at the LV Center doesn't involve us—not directly. It happened during a family group session. We sat in a wonky circle, parents next to their teenagers. There was a girl. I don't remember her name, just that she had dark hair and a sweet young face, like all the girls did when not angry, crying, or defiant. Everyone was encouraged at some point to speak, and we must have carefully shared fears, concerns, and wishes.

Maybe this girl's father was present. Maybe I only want him to be present and so have conjured him there in the chair beside hers. More likely she was alone, but that thought is too much to bear even these many years later. Someone asked the girl where her mother was, why she wasn't with us in this session or, come to think of it, in previous ones either.

Her face crumpled—a mix of pain, resignation, anguish, and sorrow. We watched as she struggled to maintain her composure, grasping for dignity. The pressure inside me to act, to hug or hold her, was enormous, but I sat still. "One too many trips to treatment, I guess," she said, resigned to the unbearable too muchness of herself.

How dare that woman, I thought.

Mind you, the shock was not in knowing that a kid could feel her mother's love was conditional.

The shock was knowing that under certain circumstances any one of us could become *that* mother. The mother who flees.

THE REAL BOTTOM

Holly, LV's director, waved me into her office; this was after Presidents' Day weekend, about ten days after I canceled the D.C. trip. I had just placed dinner in Faith's cubby, was about to dash back outside to the car.

Holly shut the door. We sat on opposite sides of her big, tidy desk. "Faith saw the nurse today," she said. They'd instituted regular body checks when the self-harming behavior began. "Her newest cuts look to be a few days old. They were really deep and probably needed stitches, but it's too late now."

"Cutssss?" I asked, elongating the *s*. "Stitches?" I forced my face into a neutral mask. I hated crying in front of the people involved in Faith's care. It made me feel ridiculous and ineffective.

"It's time for you and Theo to consider residential treatment. Her anxiety is out of control. We aren't equipped to deal with the severity of her self-harming here. Our biggest fear is that she's only fourteen. She might not be trying to kill herself, but she could easily make a mistake. We've seen it happen."

Faith's anxiety, not even an official diagnosis, had been building in advance of a family wedding planned for the holiday weekend. So many people. So much food. For several family sessions we'd attended beforehand, with Amy, we'd discussed that Faith couldn't avoid triggering situations forever, and that we hadn't gone anywhere since New Year's. We'd made a plan and had followed through, and I'd thought things had gone fine. But in light of this new information, Faith's improved mood over the weekend made a new awful kind of sense.

"She perks up after she cuts," I said.

"Yes, self-harm relieves anxiety. Frankly, she doesn't want to stop." Looking sorrowful, Holly handed me a Post-it Note. "I've written the name and phone number of the treatment center down for you. Talk to Theo about it and check the place out. It's really nice. The regular stay is four to six weeks." She stood. "I've already called my contact, and they have a bed available."

I stood, clutching my bulky purse, as if its heft would keep me from falling over. I must have looked like a deer in headlights. "We appreciate everything you've done," I heard myself say, polite as ever. *Did we, though?*

"You and Theo have some issues, but I wish that all of our parents were like the two of you."

"Thanks, I just wish it was enough."

In the car, I debated with myself. *We can't do this. We have to do this. What makes them think it'll change anything? Nothing else has. Is this really our only next step? They haven't even given the medication enough time to work. She's going to freak out.*

Suddenly, I was home with no memory of the drive. Inside, Theo's face grew red, and he punctured the air with his fingertips. "Fuck. This is so fucked. We can't leave her alone for a second."

"That'll only freak her out more." I was trying to sound calm, but my voice gave me away.

"We can't take a chance," he insisted. "They're right. One wrong move and she's seriously injured. Or worse."

I knew he was right. And they were right. But I was right too. We'd seen Faith's reactions to being tailgated: screaming, fighting, cutting. So far, that had been one of therapy's primary lessons—Faith had to make decisions for herself. Riding her ass would not help. But if I left her alone and something happened, I'd never forgive myself. Had we actually reached the place where Faith would be safer someplace other than our home?

Later that night, I waited in the car in the LV parking lot. Faith opened the door. "What'd Holly want?" she asked, sliding in.

"You have to go to residential. Everyone's really worried about you." My voice was shaking.

"Everyone needs to just leave me the fuck alone. I know what I'm doing."

I took a leap, named it. "It's not normal to cut yourself like this, Faith."

"I like it."

My fingers gripped the steering wheel. "Yeah, well, you're liking it right into a residential facility."

She went still, looked out the window. The remainder of the drive was silent.

At home, Faith stormed through the front door. I was right behind her. She ignored Theo's hello, went to her bedroom, and slammed the door.

Theo started. "She's in her—"

"I know. Jesus. I have to take my jacket off."

I walked to Faith's room, opened the door. "You need to leave your door open."

"Leave me alone. Can't you see I'm changing?"

Theo walked up behind me. "Fine," he said. "Leave your door open."

We retreated to the living room. She joined us a few minutes later.

"You need to stay in here with us," I told her.

"You guys are fucking assholes," Faith said, throwing herself onto the couch.

"Faith Yokas," Theo said.

"Stop," I said to both of them.

The snowball that had started rolling down the hill when this journey began had been collecting dirt every step of the way: terror, hurt, shock, fury, confusion, sadness. As of tonight, it had reached epic proportion and terminal velocity. There was no going back; we were screaming at each other.

She raced down the hallway. I ran right behind her, our footsteps thundering against the walls.

We ended up in her room. She grabbed a wooden box, hurled it at me. I jigged and it smashed into the door, bursting into pieces. She looked at me, went for the kill. "Why are you being such a fucking cunt?"

My vision went red.

I lunged, unsure of my intention. Faith dropped to the floor. I did too, and *thwap*—I gave her one good, hard whap on the butt. She kicked me.

"What the fuck is wrong with you?" she yelled.

Theo came to the doorway, looking concerned. "Guys," he said in his boss voice.

We froze, coming back into the moment. Faith wrapped her arms around her knees, rocked in place. I was trembling in rage. Disgusted with myself for losing control. Disgusted with my daughter as well. How dare she talk to me like that!

I ran for the phone and dialed Amy's number for two reasons. Incidents like this had to be reported to LV. And I hoped she would be able to calm Faith down, thus avoiding the need for another 911 call.

Amy answered. In breathless, staccato bursts, I said, "Faith . . . out of control . . . help."

I handed the phone to Faith. She shook her head. "You have to stop caring about me and leave me alone to do what I want."

As if. I shoved the phone in her hand. She put it to her ear, started to cry. Theo was still standing in the hallway. I sat on the edge of our bed, shaking. "Okay. Okay," Faith said, whimpering. A few minutes later, she hung up. "I'm going to sleep," she said, turning off her light.

Through her open door, the strand of multicolored Christmas lights strung along the archway cast shadows in red, green, and blue. I could see that Faith had curled up in a ball on the floor in the corner where some time ago she'd made a blanket fort—just like the ones she and her friends had built for sleepovers when she was little. Our cat, Finn, sat like a sphinx beside her, keeping watch, but I didn't trust him to let me know if a serious problem arose.

I grabbed a couple of pillows off my bed, dropped them on the hallway floor, and sat down. My gaze lingered on Faith's back. I was close enough to discern the motion of her torso as she breathed. On alert for any sign that might indicate she'd woken up.

Tears rolled down my cheeks. Phantom pain stung the palm I'd used to hit her. *Proud of yourself?* Hardly. I'd only spanked Faith one other time, when she was little. Horrified, I'd pledged never to do so again. I repositioned the pillows. My back, butt, and legs already ached. I scooched this way and that way, but there'd be no comfort tonight—the pain my penance.

Nothing, not even illness, gave Faith the right to treat me that way. But I'd overreacted. A loaded word, for sure, the c-word. But still just a word. Why couldn't I control myself? Was it because she didn't look sick? Because there'd been nothing to point to on a blood test, X-ray, or scan? Because no problematic tumor or cell or bone had been identified? No brace or cast or surgical procedure applied? I rubbed my hands, trying to make the pain go away.

That was the problem with mental illness, why nobody seemed to understand—because the person doesn't look sick.

Theo padded down the hallway. "I got it together," he whispered.

He meant the wooden box Faith had thrown. At some point, he'd gathered all the pieces and had been gluing the box back together in the kitchen, fixing what needed to be fixed. "And you'll probably need this." He handed me a mini flashlight.

Thanks, I mouthed.

"Watch out for your back down there." He headed for the living room.

I repositioned one of the pillows between my back and the wall. I heard a rustle, saw Faith move from the floor into her bed. I waited, listening. Quiet. When it felt like thirty minutes had passed—I don't know why not five minutes or ten or forty-five, but thirty seemed like a nice round number—I heaved myself up, walked to her bed. The Christmas lights weren't quite bright enough, so I shined the flashlight just close enough to her face: rosy cheeks, fluttering eyelids, steady breathing.

I repeated this pattern for the next four hours until I was certain that one more trip onto the hallway floor would break my legs. At the end of those four hours, Faith hadn't stirred once, so I finally lay down in my own bed.

I could see nothing on the horizon but blank space.

THE REALLY REAL BOTTOM

The residential treatment center was actually a converted single-story house in a neighborhood seventy-five miles south of home. In the makeshift lobby, I grabbed a tissue from the box on the chipped glass coffee table, blew my nose, and stuffed it into my purse with the other used tissues. Faith sat next to me, her arms crossed, her legs jackhammering.

Theo and I had trusted the recommendation sight unseen, but now I was unimpressed. The carpet was dirty. Outside the window sat a 7-Eleven and an auto parts store with barred windows. At home, our view consisted of the Santa Monica Mountain range and Boney Peak. Here, if Faith ran away, in every direction the city could swallow her up in ways I couldn't afford to consider.

I was signing my name over and over again on a one-inch stack of paperwork, my heart scorched. In the car, Faith had begged me not to do this. "I'm sorry, Mom. I'll do better." My knees still ached from climbing over the center console into the back seat to hold her for the remainder of the ride.

Theo chatted with the intake staff, as if this were a perfectly normal experience. Even though I'd acquiesced to this plan, I was thinking about making a break for it. But to where? We'd run out of options.

A phone rang. Keyboards clacked. A car honked. The normalcy made me want to stab someone with my pen. The meaning of each document barely registered through my tears and anguish. One document I signed gave temporary custody of Faith to the facility. If she decided to run away or injured herself, the staff needed our permission to do whatever was necessary to help her.

I struggled to keep the loose-leaf papers neat. How could a place that charged insurance one thousand dollars a day not organize with a three-ring binder? I flipped over the last page, and Theo handed the stack to the woman behind the counter. A fake potted palm tree was our only witness.

That's when someone appeared in the lobby beckoning Faith to the common area—and directing Theo and me toward the exit.

I choked back a sob. "I love you so much, babe." I wrapped my arms around her. She was stiff as a board. Tears rolled down my cheeks. I was hyperaware of the difference in our sizes—my largeness enveloping her smallness. "I hope you'll work at this. Try to get better."

I felt the soft cotton of her long-sleeved shirt, knowing what lay beneath. Before we left home, she'd cut her arm several times and Theo had bandaged the wounds.

"Don't worry, Mom," Faith said, pulling away from me. *Don't worry?* She lifted her chin. "I'll be okay."

Fluorescent lighting made her blue eyes appear gray. The stranger—an aide or nurse—opened the door that led toward the back.

"See ya later, Dad."

She walked down the corridor and out of sight.

It took every ounce of my strength to stay upright. Theo and I looked at each other, but we didn't touch in comfort. I blamed him as much as myself, and I wasn't sure at this moment that our marriage would survive.

In the car: silence.

Theo maneuvered the busy streets heading toward the 605

Freeway. I stared out the window: concrete, concrete, concrete. Leaving Faith at that place was the right thing to do, wasn't it? She'd left us no choice. I'd said *no* and *no* and *no* to residential until I couldn't, we couldn't, say no again. In my head, my fuck-ups played like an endless movie. I dug into the memory banks for something to cherish: warm beaches, vibrant blue water, sunsets, sandcastles. But each time an image bubbled up—Faith riding the purple dinosaur at our local park, Faith dancing onstage—it washed away on a wave of guilt. Not only was this illness stealing our happy present, but it was also snatching away our happy past. I leaned my forehead against the cold glass of the car window.

At home, I raced straight into Faith's room. I ripped away the blanket fort, dropped to my knees in front of her bookcase. I suspected she'd hidden some kind of self-harm stash in there, and I was determined to find it. I fanned one Warrior book and then another. *Goodnight Moon*, *The Runaway Bunny*, *Leo the Lightning Bug*, *The Kissing Hand*—favorites through various growth stages. I grabbed a batch of books off the shelf, chucked them. Grabbed another batch. Chucked those too. The pile grew. And there it was: bloody rag, Band-Aids, empty wrappers, a stained razor blade. I rocked back onto my heels. *Aha!* As if finding this evidence somehow justified sending our daughter away—as if anything could.

I ran for a trash bag, shoved everything inside, and carried it out to the bin. Maybe I was incapable of helping Faith, but I could sure as hell scrub.

Back in Faith's room, I sprayed a shelf with Windex, wiped the dust with a paper towel. I sprayed the next shelf, wiped the dust. Theo stepped in, wanted to know if I had a preference for dinner.

"In-N-Out. I want a double-double and fries."

I picked a book up off the floor, fanned through the pages looking for more contraband, and replaced it on the shelf. I fanned each additional book, returning them to the shelves. And there, again, was *The Runaway Bunny*, by Margaret Wise Brown. On the cover, a mama bunny and her baby boy bunny nestle among tall flowering grasses. The storyline revolves around the baby bunny telling his mom he's running away, and the mom's reassurances that she'll follow him, in unconditional love and support, no matter where the journey might lead.

In my mind's eye, I saw myself standing in the kitchen, those many years ago, with Faith's angry blue eyes looking up at me. "I'm leaving," she'd said. Her stuffed bunny hung limply over her arm. She'd marched out the front door, and I'd marched out behind her. Taking a cue from my dad, I'd called, "Where will you go?" She'd hesitated. I could see the gears turning. Not taking a cue from my dad, I'd said nothing further, as Faith continued down the street. I'd sat on the ledge of our front yard. She'd turned the corner, and I was calculating the distance she could go and the time it would take me to reach her when she reappeared. She walked back up the street and we hugged.

Books in order, I went to the kitchen and grabbed a bottle of chardonnay. *Moratorium over.* I popped the cork. Tonight, I no longer needed to be alert for my daughter. I didn't need to be clearheaded. My mothering duties and privileges were officially on hold. I swallowed one big sip, another, topped off the glass. I was so very tired. I headed with my glass to the couch to wait for Theo and the food and to lose myself in a TV show.

My cell phone rang. Theo and I were still watching television, surrounded by a pile of In-N-Out wrappers and bags. The wine bottle was now on the coffee table, almost empty. A social worker introduced herself, said she was from a hospital near the treatment center. "The staff nurse at the center body-checked Faith after you left and decided her newest cuts needed stitches." She meant the ones from that morning, from before we'd left for the center. No longer the surprise it should have been.

"Okay," I said. I didn't want to say much, worried the combination of wine, fatigue, and grief might cause me to slur and thereby prove that faulty mothering had landed us here.

The social worker explained that Faith wasn't doing well emotionally, as if I didn't already know that, and asked if I wanted her to go back to the treatment center after the wounds were tended.

"As opposed to?"

"She needs psychiatric care."

"That's what the treatment center is for."

"I mean hospital care."

I looked at Theo. He was listening to my end of the conversation. "We'll start with the center," I said. He nodded.

I filled Theo in about the stitches. He stared at the TV. I poured the last bit of wine from the bottle and burst into tears, again. My daughter was at a hospital with neither of her parents there for support. All the food and alcohol in the world couldn't numb this pain.

I finished the wine, cried until I no longer could. Theo kept watching TV, helpless. I wiped my nose until the tissues felt like sandpaper against my skin. My head was in a fog, felt disconnected from reality. Sleep. I needed sleep. I said goodnight to Theo, who'd watch TV for hours. I walked to Faith's room, desperate for connection to her. It was bleak, desolate. I couldn't stand it, plugged in the strand of multicolored lights that we'd unplugged before we'd left for the treatment center. "Mood lighting," I'd joked with Faith, before her only mood was dark. I walked to Faith's blinds and shut out the world.

1982

The best night of the year! The Academy Awards were about to start! I was positively panting with excitement. The glitz! The glamour! The acceptance speeches! I turned on the TV, dashed to the couch. Mom and Dad said they might watch for a while, but they didn't really care about who won.

I double-checked my supplies. *TV Guide*? Check. I carefully tore out the "Oscar Awards Close Up" page and would star the winners' names and store it later in my diary. Pen? Check. Bumpy? Check. Her cute calico face looked bored. Snacks? Nope! *Good girl.* Currently, I was back on my diet.

Let's go, let's go, let's go!

On the television, stars were strolling down the red carpet. They smiled for the cameras, waving to fans. The women looked radiant in long beaded gowns and sparkly jewelry, and the men looked dashing in their tuxedos. I desperately wanted *On Golden Pond* to win Best Picture, but *Raiders of the Lost Ark* was also nominated. Any movie a kid could watch in the theater six times and not be bored by had to be the best! But Henry Fonda! And Katharine Hepburn! The way they looked at each other in *On Golden Pond* had melted my heart. When elderly Henry admitted to Katharine that he'd gotten confused about the forest path and had hurried back to feel safe and see her pretty face, my eyes had stung. And the way she'd told him, "You're my knight in shining armor." *Ka-blam!*

A grenade of feelings had exploded in my chest. I'd tingled from head to toe. Even my ears had throbbed. And that hunky Doug McKeon—he was the reason I went back on my diet. Him and Timothy Hutton. I'd never get to act with them fat.

The orchestra music swelled, and Johnny Carson walked onto the stage. "Whoot, whoot!" I yelled. Johnny cracked jokes for a while, and then the first set of presenters walked onstage. We were off! Winners hurried out of the audience, climbed the harrowing-for-high-heels stairs, and accepted their golden statues. I cheered when their names were announced and cheered again when they said, "I'd like to thank the Academy."

I would thank the Academy, too, when I won my award. I stood up and practiced waving to the crowd, looking surprised and humble. Demure. I placed my hand on my heart, took a bow. No longer an overweight, braces-clad, pajama-wearing thirteen-year-old. I was the special one, in the spotlight.

In my fantasy, I scanned the sea of beautiful faces, the hands clapping for me. I was bedazzled, like them, skinny, like them, coifed. As a famous actress, photographers would beg to take my picture. Throngs of fans would clamor for my autograph. Sometimes I'd oblige, of course. A star must keep her supporters contented.

But sometimes I wouldn't. A star must also keep some allure, keep people wanting more. Out and about, I'd wear giant sunglasses, a floppy hat, and a scarf—drive away from the peons in my convertible with silky tails flapping impolitely in the wind.

Life would be easier when I became famous and rich. I'd have a personal chef prepare my meals, so I'd know exactly what to eat and how much. I'd have a personal exercise guru, so I'd stay thin. Most important, I'd have my choice of men, so I'd never have to pine for anyone ever again. I wouldn't do anything I didn't want to do. Burning someplace deep inside me was the need to not be ordinary. Big things lay in store for me, and I could see it all in my mind. I plopped back onto the couch.

A couple of hours later, Mom called from upstairs. "It's late. Time for bed."

"No. It isn't over yet," I said, annoyed.

I returned my attention to the screen. Sissy Spacek, her long auburn hair swept into an updo, was talking about growing up in Texas and how Oscar night was the best night of the year. "Yes, ma'am." She announced the names of the five nominees for Best Actor. "And the Oscar goes to . . ." She opened the envelope. "Henry Fonda for *On Golden Pond*." The audience and I went wild.

Jane Fonda accepted the award for her father, while I cried tears of joy.

DAY ONE

The morning after we dropped Faith off at residential, I woke up. My eyes felt like baseballs, my stomach roiling with the full force of Faith's absence landing on my chest like a boulder. I resented the sun for shining. I stared up at the soundproofing popcorn. I hated that crap. Dust had accumulated on it, twirling and twisting in the ceiling fan breeze. But it hit me: no emergency phone call had come during the night. Hadn't they said someone would check on Faith every fifteen minutes? She must be doing okay. Could I allow myself a modicum of relief?

I used the bathroom, my head pounding, grabbed my robe, and saw that Faith's bedroom door was closed. *What the fuck?* Theo must have closed it last night before climbing into bed. A closed bedroom door, a room maintained as a shrine, was the act of a parent whose child had died. I wanted to scream, "OUR DAUGHTER IS NOT DEAD!"

I shoved open the door, my heart pounding. Everything remained exactly as it had been left the prior day—a suspended animation of colored lights, closed blinds, unrumpled bed. Faith wasn't there. *Faith's gone.* My knees loosened. She wasn't in the bathroom, the living room, or anywhere else in the house. She wasn't about to go to school, see her friends, or complain about homework. We wouldn't chat, or debate, or argue. In fact, at this moment I had no idea what my fourteen-year-old daughter was doing. The center had given us a schedule, but I hadn't reviewed it yet. I stormed down the hallway.

Theo sipped coffee at the kitchen table.

"Did you close Faith's door?" I demanded.

"Yeah, I just thought—"

"Well, don't. Do not close it again." I sounded unhinged.

I ripped open the fridge, dumped creamer in my mug—the mug from Mom's place. Theo watched me yank the coffee pot from its base.

"Have a headache?" he asked.

"No," I lied.

Nerves vibrating, I plunked down across from him. With a hangover, my coffee smelled like dirt. I took a sip. Tasted like dirt too. *Faith's gone.* An eerie quiet settled around me. We gave up on her. We quit on our daughter. The thought was insistent as an alarm. I felt Theo's eyes on me. Another word from either of us could turn this conversation sideways.

"I think I'll do some work in the garage," Theo said, heading for the door.

A wide berth was the smart choice.

I wandered back to Faith's room and stood in the soft glow of the lights. I faced the bookcase, watching a vision of myself splay books across the floor, felt the same sense of cleanliness I had after each load of sullied laundry made clean. I walked to the dresser, covered in notes, trinkets, and the small stuffed Abominable Snowman, Bumble, from *Rudolph, The Red-Nosed Reindeer* I'd finally found on eBay and paid a fortune for the year she'd asked for it from Santa. And pictures: Faith in her Gator Girls soccer uniform, Theo and me in the backyard, daisies tucked behind my ears. At the bed, I extracted her pillow, hugged it to my body. Breathed in. *Damn it.* Fabric softener. Clutching the pillow to my chest, I rocked. If leaving Faith in treatment was the right decision, why did I feel so wrong?

I stayed in that position for a while, next to the bed, cradling the pillow. Finally, I replaced it, smoothed the wrinkles out of the comforter. I didn't want Theo to know I'd been here. I noticed the empty spot on top of the stuffed animal pile in the hot-pink baby doll crib where Cherry Puller had been sitting. Faith was allowed to have one stuffed animal in treatment, and she'd wanted the one from her grandmother.

I headed to the couch, where I planned to spend the rest of the day.

Four episodes of *Law & Order: SVU* later, Theo was unwrapping the foot-long Subway sandwich I'd asked him to pick up for lunch. I grabbed plates and a bag of salt and vinegar chips.

"We have to study the booklet," Theo said.

"Study?"

"We're responsible for knowing and adhering to all the rules."

I couldn't have cared less about the rules. I'd spent all morning in my pj's in front of the TV. I had no plan to get dressed. Felt like I might never want to get dressed again. My teeth weren't brushed; my hair wasn't combed. My therapist, Kim, was continuing to tell me that Faith needed to see me take care of myself, but her words didn't matter because Faith was gone, and wouldn't be back soon. We'd been told she'd likely be at treatment for at least a month.

"You go first," I said, carrying my food to the table. "I'll read it when you're done."

Between bites, Theo flipped pages. He'd loaded his half of the sandwich with a huge pile of jalapeno peppers—his secret weapon for staying healthy, looking years younger than his actual age—and was wiping sweat from his forehead with a napkin. "I'll go over it again later with a highlighter to make it easier to spot the most important information," he said. Then he handed the booklet to me.

The center had rules about everything: how long we had to wait to see our own kid for the first time, when and how to call in, when and how long we could speak, when and how long we could visit after the first time, how mail would be opened and read by someone prior to Faith. *Sounds like juvie.* Faith wasn't bad; she was sick. Why were we being treated like criminals?

I turned to the section on the center's phase system. There were five phases—pre-phase to phase four—and each one had a series of treatment objectives, restrictions, and privileges, like daily showering, not cursing, and participating in therapy. Faith would have to move through the phases in order to return home. Each phase also listed a minimum to maximum duration. After shaking potato chip dust from the bag into my mouth, I grabbed a pencil and jotted down the maximum totals for each of the five phases: twelve weeks. I dropped the pencil. No one had said anything about Faith being gone for three months.

I went to the garage. "Did you see the time frames?" I asked Theo. He was at his work bench, manually reloading ammunition to shoot targets at the range—his only hobby besides golf.

"Yeah," he said. "It's up to her how long she's there." He pulled down on the lever, seating a bullet with a case. *Ka-dunk.* "She's got to have the willingness to do the work. Did you see everything she has to do?"

I resented how rational he sounded, how calculated, how distant. I wanted him to be outraged, like me. I ignored his question, went inside, grabbed my box of tissues, and returned to the couch.

SCARIEST PHONE CALL EVER

Day two. Theo and I called Faith after lunchtime, at one o'clock, and put the phone on speaker. We waited forever for Faith to get on the line. My heart pounded and my ears actually rang.

"Hello?" Faith said.

That voice! "Hi, babe, how ya doin'?" I asked.

"Fine."

"Dad and I are both here. How are you feeling?"

"Fine."

I strained toward the phone. I needed more information, to hear her pacing and pitch. We were allotted twenty minutes for this call, and I planned to use every minute to figure out if my daughter hated me for doing this to her. If the roles were reversed, I'd hate me.

"Did you eat your lunch?" Theo asked.

Good question. We'd emphasized to Faith's new primary therapist, Dr. Amanda, that while Faith's discharge summary from the LV Center indicated she was not currently engaging in eating disordered behaviors, the new staff would have to monitor meal times to make sure Faith ate and didn't run off to purge. Without the ability to self-harm, the likelihood was high that disordered eating behaviors would reemerge—the "normal" Whac-A-Mole at play.

"Yes," she sighed.

"Was it good?" I cut in. "Is the food good there?"

"It's fine."

I was already at a loss about what else to say, just so happy to hear her voice, to have a connection through the line.

"You know we can't visit until you earn the right?" I asked.

Silence.

I felt awkward, like I was conversing with someone I just met, except this was my kid. I plowed on: "We're not trying to irritate you, but right now you're the only way we have to get information."

"Okay."

Silence.

"You sure you're okay?" I asked. *Stupid.*

"I'm fine," she snapped.

"Did you sleep okay?" I asked.

"No. They woke me up, like, every ten minutes." Protocol for kids on suicide watch. "I'm exhausted."

"They wanted to make sure you were safe," I said.

"We won't be able to talk again until Wednesday," Theo said. This was Saturday.

"Okay."

Silence.

Would we ever have an ordinary conversation again?

Theo and I glanced at one another. "Anything else?" he asked.

"Nope."

Seconds ticked by.

This call was heading nowhere. I didn't know what I'd expected, but it was more than this.

"Okay, then," Theo said.

"We'll talk when we can, I . . ." I said.

The line went dead.

". . . love you."

This place was supposed to help us, not drive the wedge deeper. We were allowed twenty minutes; the call lasted only five.

Theo removed his glasses, rubbed his eyes.

"That didn't go well," I said. "Did she sound okay to you?"

He shrugged. We sat for a minute. I walked back to the TV. Theo went back to the garage.

Later, no one had the energy to cook dinner. "What sounds good?" Theo wanted to know. After months of eschewing my favorite dinners in order to placate the eating disorder, I intended to eat what I wanted.

"Something gooey and cheesy," I said. "Italian."

I ordered the lasagna family dinner—a meal that could feed four—just for the two of us. *Leftovers*, I told myself. Yeah, right.

LOINS

I stepped out of the shower and toweled off. Today was the day. Two agonizing weeks (and more stilted phone calls) after we'd dropped Faith off at the treatment center, we were finally scheduled for our first full family session. And for Faith, I would do what I hadn't done in a while.

I slipped on real clothes, not sweats. In the mirror I saw damp hair, a ruddy complexion, and dark circles under my eyes. I was gaining more weight, and before I could stop it: *You look like shit*. As if I didn't already know that. I massaged mousse into my hair anyway, which had finally gained back some length.

Just before Mom's funeral, seven months ago now, I'd gone to her salon for a trim. My arrival there that day and the realization, *This is Lauraine's daughter*, had sent a current through the place where Mom had been going for years. The more the woman cut and the more the other women talked about my mother, telling me how much they loved and admired her, the more confused I'd felt about why my experiences didn't match what other people said. I had no memories, for example, of Mom doing things like washing, brushing, or styling my hair. No doting, period. It was Dad, I recalled, who took me for cuts. The more my hair fell on the floor, the shorter I'd told the woman to keep cutting. "Enough?" Mom's lady had finally asked, looking concerned. "A little more," I'd said. The last time my hair was that short was back before Dad moved to California, when I thought he might die. Cutting it felt like some kind of symbolic act. A ritual, but of what I wasn't sure.

I grabbed a brush and the hair dryer, bent over, short strands reaching for the floor, and hit it with heat. Somewhere along the line, a hairstylist had told me that drying hair upside down adds volume, so that's how I did it. I hung upside down, blood rushing to my head, strands flying every which way until I got a little dizzy. I levered upright, raking my scalp with the brush to smooth out the volume's excess poufiness, the dryer whirring its white noise.

Next, spilling the contents of my makeup bag onto the counter, I pumped primer into my hand and smoothed it over my face. When Faith was growing up, I'd tried to be careful not to disparage my body out loud—*gross, disgusting, ugly.* And I'd tried not to cast a critical eye at my reflection, raise an eyebrow over the size of my butt. I'd hidden those self-judgments behind silence camouflaged with a cheerful wink and a smile. Hadn't I?

Concealer, eyeliner, mascara. Powder, blush, eyebrow pencil. Compared to Faith's self-harming, thinking about my body image issues and low self-esteem felt shallow. But it wasn't shallow. Our bodies were, in fact, ground zero. Every girl and woman I'd ever known, even the prettiest ones, going back almost as far as I could remember—Mom, aunts, cousins, friends, friends' moms, friends' cousins, coworkers, acquaintances, strangers, and, of course, almost every female character on television and in movies—had obsessed openly about their bodies, had vilified, denounced, defamed, belittled, condemned, and complained about their body's size, shape, inadequacies, and imperfections.

Now, I had to add my daughter to that list, and if I'd had the opportunity to know either of my grandmothers, they'd probably be on the list too. I could literally think of only one woman I'd met at a function, a year or two before Mom died, whom I'd believed when she said she never gave a single thought to what she weighed.

Of course, she was thin.

Lip gloss, hair spray, topped with a spritz of vanilla-y perfume. I thought about little Faith, twirling around in her exersaucer, watching me style my hair and apply makeup. And Faith, not that long ago, watching, the way I'd watched my mother, who, I assumed, had watched her mother.

Okay. Hair? Check. Makeup? Check. Not perfect, of course, but I felt better about myself for having made the effort. Faith would never know the full extent of my struggles, and that was the point.

At the treatment center, Faith's new primary therapist, Dr. Amanda, called Theo and me into her office. She wore jeans with Birkenstocks. Long, curly black hair streaked with gray framed her face. During Faith's initial assessment, we'd learned that Dr. Amanda was new to the facility, only recently having passed her licensing exams. I wondered if she had the necessary experience for a case as serious as Faith's.

Theo and I settled into the '70s-era couch. Without preamble, Dr. Amanda blurted out, "Faith's not making much progress."

Nothing like a little negativity to get the ball rolling.

Faith walked in then, and I launched myself at her like a rocket. Was that blood on her jeans?

"You look pretty," she said, hugging me. "You smell good too."

I squeezed her so hard she squeaked.

As Faith hugged Theo, I took a good look at her. She looked like herself, sort of. Her old smile, the one before depression, had been intense and bright. The smile she was attempting now looked like an effort. Her hair was clean, but her eyes weren't right. The corners drooped. She looked depleted, as if the energy had been sucked out of her body. The difference may have been subtle to everyone else, but not to me.

Dr. Amanda plunged in. “I can feel tension between the two of you.” She was looking at Theo and me. “Did anything big happen between you when all of this began?”

I sighed. Theo crossed his legs. Strains in our marriage, like differences in parenting styles and communication skills, had been a topic of conversation in the therapy we’d attended since the very beginning. Of course the stress of Faith’s illness had exacerbated those issues, but they predated Faith’s illness. So while it was true that things between us were worse than they’d been in a long while, I was out of patience with this line of questioning. And Faith wasn’t oblivious. She knew her illness had impacted our relationship, which made her feel even worse. A discussion about our marriage, in family session, would be too open to misinterpretation by her. Besides, our reactions to what was happening were our responsibility, not hers. We were there to lift her up.

“No,” I said. “Our marriage has had its ups and downs, sure, but the big thing we’ve been through recently was my mom’s death.” I glanced at Faith. She was already frowning.

“Faith mentioned that was part of the catalyst to stop eating,” Dr. Amanda said. I sat up. This was the first time an outright, spoken connection between the two events had been made, and I wanted to explore the idea further, to see if we could get closer to understanding what one had to do with the other and how to untangle them. But Dr. Amanda had her own agenda. Switching topics, she said, “Faith’s on a seventy-two-hour hold.”

“What do you mean?” Theo asked.

Dr. Amanda explained that Faith had scratched herself with a staple she found on the floor and with her nails. “She’s stuck in phase one until the hold is over.” The doctor paused for dramatic effect.

I doubted threats would motivate Faith. They hadn’t in the past, and, in general, they seemed like a piss-poor treatment strategy. I didn't understand behavior modification tactics—not self-harming leading to positive consequences and self-harming leading to negative consequences—and punishment as "treatment" for mental health conditions. Dr. Amanda continued: "I'm really frustrated because she's not doing the work."

Theo and I looked at each other. We'd been down this road twice, feared what came next. The mental health professional assigned to help us would claim they no longer could.

"Are you already ready to quit on her too?" Theo asked.

"Yeah, I want them to quit," Faith said. "I want to kill myself."

Theo sniffed. I knew he wouldn't cry. Never did. But I started to cry. So much for my makeup. I was desperate to find out what Dr. Amanda was actually doing to help Faith. What she expected would have changed after two measly weeks when we'd been at this for seven months. And what, in this place's view, "doing the work" even meant. Before I could say anything, Dr. Amanda leaned forward.

"Theo, can you tell Faith how you'd feel if she killed herself?"

Faith stiffened. My arms and legs went limp. I stared at Dr. Amanda. The gray in her hair looked brittle. What kind of question was that? What words could ever do justice to the aftermath of a child's suicide? I looked at Theo. He looked as shocked as I felt. I held my breath, worried that his response would veer off course, confusing Dr. Amanda, hurting Faith, and disappointing me.

"It would be the worst possible thing that could happen," Theo said, grimly.

Good. Simple.

Then he let out a throaty little laugh.

"Do you find this funny?" Dr. Amanda asked.

Theo tugged at the bill of his ball cap. He was not used to being challenged. "No, I do not. You don't know this about me, but my first wife died in my arms." Theo's voice cracked—and just like that, there she was, again. Nineteen years after her death: Theo's first wife, Vivienne.

I cried harder, the familiar ache of inadequacy exploding inside me. I stared at my lap.

"Vivienne was a frail nothing of the beautiful bride I'd once had. My mother died in my arms too." Theo turned to Faith. "All of this would be nothing compared to the loss of you, because you come from my loins."

Ugh. Loins?

Faith started to cry, pulled away from me. "I love you guys, but I can't handle this." She bolted out the door.

"That's the first real emotion I've seen out of her," Dr. Amanda said.

Is that what this was about—a choreographed attempt to get Faith to emote something "real"?

Disgusting.

On the drive home, passing the concrete and the barred windows, I worried about Faith, of course, and Dr. Amanda. *Awful*. I wondered if we could switch therapists. I wondered what the actual plan was to help Faith, and why Dr. Amanda had ignored the clue about my mother's death. Yes, Faith was there to participate, again, in individual and group therapies, and to do chores and earn privileges, but I thought, again, that if a structure designed for behavior modification was going to help, it would have by now. Everything about this process felt wrong. I needed a distraction. My brain was reeling from the session and, after so many years, still, from hearing Vivienne's name. I turned up the radio, hoping for relief that would never come.

Theo and I never discussed Vivienne. Early on, sensing my insecurity, he'd say reassuring things like, "I don't think about the past," and "You're the one I love now," and "You make me want to be a better man." I believed what he said because Theo was a man of his word. But because I knew the history, I knew that Theo had left out a couple of details with Dr. Amanda. Over an eighteen-month span, Theo had lost his first wife and his mother, yes, but also his father, and last but not least, the coup de grâce, his dog of fourteen years. Then he met me, escaping grief and death by falling in love and sweeping me off my feet.

Silence was an unspoken rule that I'd never questioned or broke. But because we'd never brought Vivienne into the open, she'd lived in my mind. In there, I used to picture Theo lying on a hospital bed next to his blond-haired, blue-eyed bride, his strong arms wrapped around her frail body. The way he must have stroked her hair, spread like a halo on the antiseptic pillow. They whispered words I could never hear. I'd never shared my secret thoughts with Theo. And sixteen years of marriage later, for reasons I couldn't understand, I'd been unable to completely move on from the comparison only I was making. Vivienne was dead and gone. Why couldn't I stop comparing myself to a ghost? And now, all over again, I wondered if I'd ever stop feeling like sloppy seconds.

At home, the light on the answering machine was blinking. Dr. Amanda had called to say she'd checked on Faith in the common area and she'd seemed "happy as a lark." I stabbed the delete button, headed for the couch.

1987

I was home from college on a break, at Mom's place. Must have been my sophomore year, because the house on the lake was long since sold, the divorce was in the works, if not final, and she'd moved from an apartment to a small condo. I hadn't forgiven her for leaving Dad, wasn't sure I ever would. And the way she'd left him. Waiting until after they'd purchased a small home together in another state where "they'd" decided to retire only to tell him she changed her mind. He'd had no choice but to follow through, on his own, leaving behind his whole life.

We were at Mom's condo getting ready to go out. She was in the tiny bathroom putting the final touches on her makeup. I was watching her stare at herself in the mirror, wand mascara onto her eyelashes. My mother was objectively an attractive woman. She'd lost some weight ("I'm back on the market!"), was already dating. I was having a hard time wrapping my head around their diametrically opposed reactions to the split: Dad's utter emotional deterioration, her blasé laissez-faire attitude. I mean, even though it was her decision, they'd shared twenty years together. And me. Was there nothing to be sad about?

Sometimes I wondered if my mother was capable of feeling anything.

To me, looking at Mom in the mirror, at this moment, I could only see the imperfections: crooked teeth, giant mole, a few gray hairs. Furious, unconscious to the true kernel of my rage—Dad's despair, the apparent farce of my childhood, the lies—I aimed instead for her face. I knew there'd be a cost, but I was prepared to pay.

"Why do you do that? I asked, wondering if her mother had done it that way.

In the mirror, her eyes met mine. "Do what?"

"Make that stupid shape with your mouth?"

I mimicked the sort of O shape that formed every time she applied mascara. I'd always hated how she did that. Why couldn't she put mascara on like a normal person, like the rest of us? She had to act all haughty, do it the way I imagined a movie star might. That's what I usually thought, anyway. Now, I was just pissed.

She frowned, her eyes narrowed. "I don't know. That's just what my mouth does."

I walked away.

In the condo's only bedroom, I stood in front of the closet trying to decide what to wear. I had fewer options, as some of my clothes no longer fit, again. I'd gained the requisite "freshman fifteen," along with a few more divorce pounds. Dad's shock and tears the previous summer had fueled the flames of my insatiable hunger. I grabbed a wool skirt and was shimmying into it when I heard a cluck.

Mom, framed by the bathroom doorway, was watching me, her nose wrinkled. "You really need to lose some weight," she said. As if I didn't already know that.

There was no sense in arguing. "I know," I said, hoping to shut down the burning core of my shame, instantly feeling the same disgust Mom did.

Mom walked away. I sucked in my gut, zippered the skirt. It always boiled down to the same bottom line. Achievements, like my induction in high school into the National Honor Society, winning the John Philip Sousa Band Award for my leadership, dependability, loyalty, and cooperation, and getting accepted to one of my top choice universities, were of no consequence. Nothing would outshine the disappointment of my body.

GARBAGE BAG

Hundreds of thousands of Catholics were crammed into St. Peter's Square in Rome, waving flags, praying, shouting, crying tears of joy. Waiting to catch a glimpse of the newly elected pontiff, Cardinal Jorge Bergoglio, Pope Francis. Six days after that disappointing family session with Dr. Amanda, I was glued to the TV, astounded per usual by the Catholic Church's obsession with pomp and circumstance, the offensive opulence.

The television announcers were debating what might be different about Pope Francis, compared to his predecessors, due to his humble background. How early exposure to poverty might shape his papacy. In my view, the chances that one man could change what had for millennia been broken seemed at best abysmal.

The phone rang. My heart skipped, and I raced to answer it.

"It's Dr. Amanda. I'm sorry, but I have bad news."

"Is Faith okay?" I held my breath.

"Oh, yes." I released my breath. "But I called the mobile team to come and evaluate her. She's cutting a lot. They just arrived and are assessing whether or not she should go to the hospital."

She meant the psych ward. My stomach dropped.

"She's not safe, and the hospital will stabilize her. I'll call you when I know more." With that, the line went dead.

I filled Theo in, and we agreed we'd drive straight to the hospital if Dr. Amanda called with the news we'd dreaded.

I threw on clothes, waited on the couch, watching the news and remembering my only experience with inpatient psychiatric care—a college field trip for abnormal psych class. One of my classmates was a devilishly handsome guy, and his mere presence had caused two of the female patients to vie for his attention. They'd almost come to fisticuffs. Orderlies had swooped in to break it up, and we were ushered out. For a long time, I wondered what happened to the women after we left. I wondered what happened behind the locked doors of a psych ward. Were we about to find out?

Within the hour, Dr. Amanda called to inform me that Faith was being transported to College Hospital. Theo and I practically ran to the car. Halfway through the drive, I finally reached a ward nurse who let me know that Faith had arrived at the hospital with nothing but the clothes on her back—no pj's, toothbrush, undies. *Figures.* Inept Dr. Amanda. Had she cared even one iota? I called the treatment center and said we'd stop by to pick up the things Faith needed.

When we got there, Dr. Amanda called us into her office. "I'm really sorry," she said, reclining in her chair, "but Faith won't be able to come back."

Dread gripped my chest. *No, no, no.*

"She's cutting too much, and she's just too much of a liability," Dr. Amanda added, refusing to meet my gaze.

I couldn't speak. *Liability?*

The word hung in the air. I was trying to think, my brain scrambling to make sense of a treatment center refusing to treat someone who needed help. Faith being jammed into the back of an ambulance, carted off to someplace else she'd never been before. More strangers. More rules. Anonymous in the system. This was help?

"What'd she get ahold of?" Theo asked.

Dr. Amanda squirmed. "One of the new girls smuggled in razor blades sewn into the lining of her teddy bear." The way she said it implied that the girl had been happy to share. "The nurse found four deep cuts on Faith's hip during body check."

I had one fully formed, crystal-clear thought: *You are rejecting her for the very reason you accepted her.*

Dr. Amanda handed me a piece of paper. "These are names of some treatment centers, mostly out of state because they can handle treatment differently there—lock the kids in, keep them safer. They're really good. We recommend that you send Faith to one for at least a year, maybe eighteen months. She needs more treatment than anyone here can provide."

Lock kids in? A year? The idea of one month away from my child was more than I could bear, and now Dr. Amanda wanted me to consider twelve months? In another state? My vision blurred.

Dr. Amanda stood. She had no more help to provide, no further guidance. We were on our own. Again.

"Sorry it didn't work out."

I wanted to tell her what I thought of her sorries. She had failed at her only job: curing Faith.

I refused to appear weak, so I did nothing but walk out the door.

In the lobby, I found Faith's suitcase next to a black, thirty-gallon garbage bag that contained most of her stuff.

A garbage bag. That's what they think of us.

While I dragged Faith's stuff to the car, Theo finalized paperwork. I rummaged through the suitcase, looking for clean clothes to take to the hospital. From the suitcase's interior state of affairs, it seemed the person who'd "packed" had done nothing more than dump Faith's dirty laundry in and zipper it closed.

I pulled a few items out, bloody. Still, I refused to consider that Dr. Amanda was right to send Faith away. Rummaging some more, I found a few clean things, and Theo and I headed for the hospital.

Driving away, I was gripped by the sensation that I was forgetting something important. I was tired, scared, confused, couldn't think straight. What was it? Not Faith. She was at the hospital. Not her suitcase. It was in the trunk with the garbage bag.

"Cherry Puller!" I screamed, flinging my arms wide. "We forgot Cherry." I burst into tears, again, and Theo turned the car around.

The woman who handed him to me said they'd forgotten him because he'd been locked in the storage closet, confiscated with other stuffed animals after the "incident."

THE WARD

Beyond the adolescent psychiatric ward's heavy automated doors, our small group of family members was bottlenecked before a windowed enclosure that appeared more military checkpoint than nurses' station. An hour or two after Dr. Amanda had told us that Faith couldn't return to the treatment center, the costumes of the sentries, green scrubs—or, worse, ones decorated in Disney characters—didn't deceive me. The gatekeepers didn't carry walkie-talkies or nightsticks, but their syringes, hidden out of sight and nearby, were filled with liquid submission.

I told myself that their presence was as much for my safety as the patients', but the thought did little to relieve me of my anxiety. Still, I didn't question their authority. I needed what this place offered, and it was time for me to admit that Faith needed it too.

When it was my turn, I signed my name into the logbook. A nurse motioned for me to hand over Faith's clothes. "We check everything," he said. "You'd be surprised what you can use to hurt yourself."

Theo stopped at the nurses' station to ask questions, unable to quite believe there were no answers. I didn't want to talk to anyone, so I went straight to the adolescent ward's small waiting room and settled down. I would wait as long as it took.

This hospital's youth services wing was for co-ed youth ages thirteen to seventeen, but you wouldn't know it by looking around. There wasn't a single splash of color in the sea of beige—a lack of vitality that made me morose. I knew from grad school that an involuntary hold usually lasted for three days. Three days to decide what was next for Faith, our family, and I wondered, again, what could change in so little time.

Patients and families kept arriving, but I made eye contact with no one. I didn't smile or acknowledge them. I couldn't. I knew Faith was where she needed to be for safety reasons, and, at the same time, I couldn't shake the feeling that this was the last place we belonged.

Except . . . here we were.

A young man, wearing a hospital ID bracelet, entered the waiting room and started pacing. He looked angry, ready to blow. I was about to move closer to the nurses' station when a girl sitting by herself in the corner caught my eye. Something about the way she was hunched over in her hospital gown and socks, her shoulders rounded under a tangled mess of black hair. It wasn't Faith. Unnaturally still, she stared straight ahead. I wanted to throw protective arms around her, hold her hand. My gaze landed on her eyes, which were completely dark. No sparkle. No hint of emotion. Where were her parents? I looked around. No one was heading her way.

Suddenly, the angry boy charged out of the waiting room toward the exit. Next came a loud crash and there he was, splayed out on the floor with a scattering of medical supplies. An orderly had tackled him—escape foiled. *Nice try, kid.* Part of me wished he'd made it out.

The orderly led the angry boy away. The dark-eyed girl remained, and I remembered the question my therapist had recently asked, in reaction to my update about the transition to residential: "What happens if Faith's not okay?" Kim meant in the long run. I'd immediately changed the subject, unable to consider

Faith not getting better. But in the hospital, I was confronted by the possibility that Faith might not improve any time soon. *What if?* I shivered, wondering if this forlorn girl was a sign of our future, if her past made this present somehow make sense.

Lellow. Elphalant, my mind imagined hearing little Faith say. And the way she would greet the day: *The sun's up! The sun's up!* Her smiling face, upstretched arms. Her hair in the sun, brown with hints of auburn and gold. The way wearing green made her blue eyes pop. The way the ocean terrified and exhilarated her until the two blended into love. I saw Theo, carrying his shovel onto the beach. How many times had he dug a giant hole, for her and anyone who wanted to join her, to play in? He dug and he dug. Down below the dry sand to the cool, wet sand. Down so far that water would leech into the bottom. Always filling it back in before we left. Me watching her and her friends, tiny feet and then bigger ones chasing the waves, playing tag on the sand, flaring out their towels, and making castles and forts. Cuddling: on the couch, in bed, at the movies. All those rising curtains.

Faith barreled into the room, straight toward me, her eyes full of defiance. "I'm not even suicidal," she said by way of a greeting. Relieved, I turned my back on the dark-eyed girl. "I just said that to fit in."

Faith's red shirt was stained with makeup, and I didn't recognize the jeans. A hospital bracelet was clamped around her wrist. She sat but was in constant motion—her legs jackhammering, arms flighty. Anxiety coursed through her like an electric current.

"I want to go back to treatment and recover with my friends," she said.

"That decision was taken out of our hands," I said firmly. "Dr. Amanda told you it was up to you. That you needed to stop cutting or she would do this."

"I don't want to be here," she said, pounding her fist into her thigh. "This is all that girl's fault, anyway. The one who gave me the razor."

She was blaming someone else. "Faith, there will always be people who are a bad influence on you." Then I surprised myself by repeating words I'd heard Theo, Mona, and Amy say: "You have to take responsibility for your own actions."

She slouched, took a long look at the surroundings: reinforced glass around the nurses' station, out the window a barbed wire–topped fence, the dark-eyed girl, who still sat motionless in her chair. Her eyes welled. "All I want to do is cuddle with you. I don't even want to cut anymore. Am I ever going to be able to come home?"

My heart leaped at the words "cuddle" and "home." I scooted my chair closer, wrapped my arm around her. She let me. "I sure as hell hope so."

"There's a razor hidden in my bookcase," she said, looking at the floor.

"I found it. Thanks for telling me, though, that means a lot."

Theo, finished with the paperwork, sat down next to us. "Hi, dollface," he said to Faith. His efforts toward a smile looked as strained and unnatural as his posture. He hated hospitals, said so whenever the word came up. After the amount of time he'd spent inside one watching his wife and mother die, he'd vowed never to set foot in one again. Yet here he was. We may have been at odds, but we were side by side caring for Faith.

"Hey, whose pants are those?" I asked Faith, hoping to lighten the mood. It worked.

"My new roommate's," she said, smiling. "I can't believe I fit in these; she's a bikini model!"

The three of us looked at each other, officially out of safe, mundane conversation topics. Theo and I weren't allowed to meet the other kids or go to Faith's assigned room. There was no television, and I didn't want a Styrofoam cup of warm water from the lone plastic jug on the counter. To keep my mind off the dark-eyed girl, who was still sitting across from me and still alone, I tried to imagine Faith living in another state, decided immediately that if it came to that, I'd move, too, for the duration of treatment. Get a job nearby, if necessary. Mama bunny hot on her baby bunny's trail. If, and this was a huge if, we could find the right place.

The PA system announced the end of visiting hours. "You need anything?" I asked, standing.

"No. I'm not even allowed to have a pencil or write in a journal."

I guessed that explained how the hospital "stabilized" things: no access to anything, at all. No wonder the stay was only three days. I couldn't imagine sitting in this drab place day after day with nothing to do but therapy. But at least we could visit our daughter every day for ninety minutes. Theo hugged Faith. Then I did. Every time I had to walk away, I had to force my arms to let go.

"We'll be back tomorrow," Theo said. And there it was again, that gruesome hospital smile.

"Try to relax and cooperate, okay?" I said. "I saw some kid get tackled a little while ago. I don't want you to be next."

SO MANY HURTING KIDS

The next morning, I walked past Faith's empty room—door open, colored lights on, blinds closed, Cherry Puller nestled on the bed awaiting her return. I knew how he felt. Three weeks. Faith had been gone for three weeks, and I was sort of starting to get used to the waiting, to how everything stayed the same day after day. The quiet. Theo and I had made the house as safe as we could. To return, Faith needed to find safety inside herself. And to do that, she needed new ways to cope.

I was trying to understand the reasoning behind behavior modification, but this was starting to feel like a chicken/egg situation. What was more important? Behavior change or thought change? Could the two actually be pulled apart? Weren't both an oversimplification of the incredibly complex dynamics between genetics, biology, and environment, including how Theo and I had parented Faith, my mother's death, and who knew what else? What would healing actually entail, and how would we know it had begun?

Coffee in hand, I sat down at my computer with the list of out-of-state facilities Dr. Amanda had given me. The hospital psychiatrist was supposed to call with an update on Faith's status. Each hour hurtled us closer to the three-day deadline—my race against time had never been more real than now. Hanging from the knob of a door on my desk was a clay heart Faith had crafted in third grade, at the center her school picture inside a small square window. To the ribbon it hung by, I'd affixed years' worth of soccer and softball photo pins. There she was, over and over again, holding a soccer ball or softball bat, her hair of varying lengths, all crinkly-eyed, dimple-cheeked, and toothy-smiled. Why her? Why us? Why anyone?

A couple of hours later, I had a dry throat and my temples were throbbing. My cell phone rang, the screen registering a call from the hospital. My chest burst with anxiety. I swiped to accept. A hospital psychiatrist introduced himself, said he was treating Faith.

"Is she okay?" I asked, holding my breath.

"Oh, yes," he said. I exhaled. "Great kid," the doctor added.

"I think so."

"I'd like to change her medication. There's a different one I prefer, and I need you to sign off."

"That's fine," I said. I didn't feel like we had a choice, and still hoped something would ease her symptoms. "And so you know," I added, "I'm making a bunch of calls trying to figure out what's next, but I'm not having much luck so far. What happens if we don't have a plan at the end of the seventy-two hours?"

"Don't worry about that. She can stay here until you figure it out."

My relief was tempered by knowing "she can stay" had so far meant until our health insurance company said Faith's coverage was used up or until a low-level administrator got tired of fighting for more time. As if fighting for our daughter's mental health wasn't hard enough, each step of the way we also had to fight with the insurance company to pay the bills, fight to prove she still needed treatment, fight about where she could or should go. We paid a small fortune every month to have quality PPO insurance. The process and how we were treated, during the worst time of our lives, was unconscionable. I bet the company accountants figured people would just give up. Bastards.

No price tag was too high for Faith's well-being, and even with good health insurance, the money I got from Mom's life insurance policy—one hundred thousand dollars—was dwindling. What would we do, I worried again, if it ran out? I put the thought out of my mind.

Four more hours and at least a dozen phone calls later, I had a full-blown headache and more information but no answers. For instance, I knew there were a lot of sick teens in our country. The treatment center in Nevada, along with centers in Utah, Illinois, and Indiana, had a four-to-six-week wait list. I had to wonder, with that many children needing help, where the actual line for "sick" began or ended. "Sick" was just another label.

How many thousands or tens of thousands or hundreds of thousands of people does it take to blur the edges of normalcy's bell curve? When does "strange" or "unusual" behavior, even if it's scary, become an "ordinary" symptom of a particular malady? Did applying a particular word hurt more than help?

Two of the out-of-state "treatment" centers refused to accept self-harming clients. Ones that did treat self-harm wouldn't accept people who weren't "buying in" to getting well. Once admitted, Faith would get only one chance, maybe two chances, to stop harming herself before she'd be discharged. Again.

I rubbed my lower back, circled my ankles. I'd been sitting without a break for hours. These days my only so-called exercise consisted of walks between the house and car and the car and treatment center or hospital. I noticed the clock: 3:10 p.m. My heart skipped. Right now, a line of vehicles was waiting to turn into the circular drive of Faith's middle school. Parents cursing, honking, cutting each other off. Not me. All around town, kids were about to eat a snack, do homework, and text with friends. Not Faith. I slammed the computer shut, no better equipped to understand our next step than I had been that morning.

"How would we keep her safe for a four-to-six-week wait?" Theo demanded later the same day. We were on our way to the hospital for our visit, and I was updating him with my findings from the afternoon.

"I guess we'd have to figure it out," I said, watching as we zoomed by the golf course.

"What if she gets kicked out of another facility? What happens to her then?"

"I have no idea, but I doubt it would be good for her fragile psyche."

"And how far away is too far?" he asked.

"There is no 'too far' for the right place, Theo."

"How are we going to make this decision?"

"I don't know," I replied. "We need more information."

"You're the one with the therapy degree. Why can't you figure this out?"

At this, I sucked in a breath. "I cannot believe you just said that to me," I said.

Theo kept his eyes on the road. He neither apologized nor retracted his words. When he finally spoke, all he said was, "Well?"

I stared out the window: rolling hills, shopping center, Erewhon sign. Sure, he was scared. I knew that. But so was I. Kim and I had spoken about my habit of confronting Theo when he was insensitive toward me, the way he would ignore or twist my words, and my tendency to then drop the matter while adding every unresolved infraction to a growing list of resentments. I could feel Kim urging me to use an "I" statement—something like, "I feel very hurt by your implication that I'm not smart enough to help Faith." But I didn't. Partly because I knew Theo thought there was nothing wrong with what he'd said. And partly because I half thought he was right—I *should* have known what to do. My only comfort was that no one else with a degree, and we'd met lots of degrees—MS, MFT, LCSW, PhD, RN, MD—knew what to do either.

Ninety minutes later, at the hospital, we locked my purse and Theo's wallet in the trunk. Hospital policy. Faith was wearing a different shirt but the same jeans. The dark-eyed girl wasn't in the waiting area, and I refused to consider what her absence might mean. Otherwise, this visit was like the prior day's visit: Faith wondering what would happen next, for which I had no answer, and the three of us attempting mundane small talk.

When the PA announced the end of visitation, we stood. "By the way," Faith said. "I got my period back today."

"That's good news," I said, clapping my hands.

Theo sighed in relief.

"I guess," she said, walking away.

Then I thought, *Something normal and it's still about blood.*

BATTLE ARMOR, KIT UPDATE

Lotion
Eye drops
Treatment document
A Bright Red Scream, by Marilee Strong

WHAT'S MY GUT GOT TO DO WITH IT?

"I don't trust anyone," I said to Kim.

Two days after Dr. Amanda had sent Faith to the hospital and the morning after Faith got her period, I was filling Kim in—the garbage bag, the "liability" comment, the hours of phone calls, and my refusal to delegate any of the research to Theo. "I don't understand," I said. "What's the point of treatment if it's only for people who want to get better? How many people start out wanting to get better? What about the rest of us?"

I thought about my struggle with postpartum depression, how I hadn't even understood what was happening until I was already coming out of it, and my grad school practicum, providing supervised therapy to real clients who often looked confused at the mention of a diagnosis, and the way Faith would say that Theo and I had "the problem," not her. "Most people, especially starting out, lack insight into their mental health issues," I added, saying what an experienced therapist would already know.

"What's your gut tell you?" Kim asked.

"What do you mean? About what?"

"No one knows your daughter better than you do. You're the expert on Faith."

I'm the Faith expert? I'd always felt this to be true in a Tylenol or Motrin sort of way, back before Faith's mental health crisis. But now? What if Kim was right? What if Theo and I had placed too much trust in the system, not enough in ourselves? No one was more invested in Faith's well-being than we were, than I, her mother, was. *I'm the Faith expert*. Clearly, there was no one "right" course of action for Faith's healing. So far, I had not considered that my opinion mattered most for the most beautiful reason: the essence of Faith—her skin, bones, blood, heart, and brain—had blossomed inside of me. I'd nurtured her long before anyone else could and would do so long after others might fall by the wayside. No one shared the bond I had with Faith, no matter how tenuous that bond currently felt. The opinion I needed to respect was my own.

"What's your gut say?" Kim asked, again.

At home, feeling somehow empowered, I reorganized my to-do list with vigor. If there was one skill I'd mastered during my years working in the entertainment business, it was organization. Not necessarily the most experienced or even skilled production manager, I'd made up for the deficit by working harder and longer.

I called every clinician we'd seen and more we'd never met. I repeated our story to administrators at seven more facilities in three more states. I jotted down copious notes on treatment modalities, philosophies, and core values. I studied frequently asked questions and testimonials and checked accreditation.

No one had an answer. Everyone had an opinion.

You have to treat the eating disorder first. You have to treat the self-harm first. Cutting isn't as bad as you think. A group setting will make her worse. She'll only get better in a group setting. Twelve-step ideologies fit well with the treatment of your daughter's problems. Twelve-step ideologies don't fit with the treatment of your daughter's problems. Bringing her home would be a management nightmare and could send you over the edge. Bringing her home is the best thing you could do. It sounds like your daughter's case has been mismanaged from the beginning.

If we've mismanaged Faith's case since the beginning, I thought, *I'm powerless to change it now.* And what an awful thing to tell a parent struggling to help their child. What could I do now about the past?

Six hours later, all I knew, still, was that each place was wrong for its own reason—the wait list was too long or the stay was too short, the cost was too much or the services weren't enough. I felt like saying to someone, "This is too hard. You do it." But there was no one else. And I would not do to Faith what that mother of the girl from the LV Center had done. No way. Faith would not end up in a group session somewhere talking about how I'd quit on her. Quit on us.

My phone rang—the hospital social worker assigned to Faith's case. We chatted for a second about what a great kid he thought Faith was. Again, I agreed. "Yes, she's the only one who doesn't seem to know."

Then he dropped the bomb. "I'll need your decision by Monday," he said. "I want to discharge her on Tuesday."

It was Friday. I had three days. Again.

Later that day, I was in the bedroom, dressing for visiting hours. I squeezed toothpaste from the tube, peppered myself with questions: *Has Faith progressed enough for us to facilitate treatment from home with new clinicians? Has she progressed at all? Not likely. There hasn't been enough time. But she does want to come home—does she want it enough to stop hurting herself? Is there any amount of talking or workbook pages that can solve these problems? Will her recent medication change help or hurt?*

At the LV Center, we'd discussed a safety plan—a detailed description of Faith's responsibilities to avoid destructive behavior and the actions we'd take if she hurt herself—but we'd sent her to residential before giving it a chance.

Will a safety plan be enough to forestall tragedy? To scare her into submission? What kind of solution is that, anyway?

My brain throbbed.

Cut to the chase.

I doused my face with water, dried off. When I shook clean the Etch A Sketch of other peoples' opinions and the prevailing rhetoric, I saw one question: Would Faith be better off hundreds, thousands, of miles away with a new set of strangers, or would she be better off coming back home to try again with the people who loved her most?

Who would take better care of my daughter? Them or me?

In the car now, again, green grass and trees of the golf course whizzing by, I told Theo we were on our own. He knew about the social worker's call, the deadline. "No one knows what to do," I said. "And no one can say what Faith may or may not do." I paused, the weight of my words—their implication—sinking in. I fiddled with the air conditioner vents, unable to adjust the flow how I wanted it, gave up. Finally, I knew what my gut was telling me. "What if I said I want to bring Faith home? I feel like we gave the system its chance, and it didn't do any better than we did."

"I think you're right," Theo said. "They've done a crap job so far."

A meeting of our minds. Refreshing.

"We can't say anything to her yet," I said. "I have to make a bunch of calls this weekend to get everything in place."

"And I'll get something to lock up the knives and stuff."

I opened my notebook—I carried it everywhere—and started a weekend to-do list. Some people would think it was wrong, dangerous even, to bring Faith home, but this decision couldn't be worse than the one we'd made to send her away. Part of trusting myself included trusting my ability to help formulate a workable plan and identify if the plan started falling apart. At a time when nothing made sense, Faith coming home was one thing that did.

THE COMEUPPANCE

Saturday morning. Faith was still in the hospital. I parked at the strip mall near home, in front of Weight Watchers, cut the engine. *Back again*, I thought, grimly.

Inside, there was a long line of folks checking in. This Weight Watchers looked like all the other ones. I recognized familiar faces behind the counter. By the whiteboard, Dolly. I'd stepped into a time warp—everything as it had been every time I rejoined the program since Faith was six months old.

I caught Dolly's eye, waved. She smiled, waved back. She never looked surprised or disappointed to see me again—the neutral mask of a practiced therapist. I lined up to weigh and pay.

Ahead of me, men and women kicked off every extraneous ounce—shoes, purses, watches, wallets, jackets, anything—before stepping onto the digital scales, into the sweaty footprints of the person before. Nowadays, a computer printer spit out a label with the date and time, your name, current weight, daily point allotment, and the plus or minus in pounds and ounces of the current weight compared to the previous week's weight. No numbers were announced out loud; the receptionists just affixed the label into each person's weight record, took payment, and ushered us on.

I awaited my turn, dreading the comeuppance I was sure to face from the last eight months of overeating. All the clichés ran through my mind: time to *pay the piper*, *face the music*, *take my medicine*, *bite the bullet*, and, Dad's favorite, *shit or get off the pot*. I was wearing extra-large thin fabric exercise pants, but somewhere along the line, getting ready to visit Faith, I'd had to dig my way to the back of my closet for size 16 jeans—a size larger than normal. I doubted my ability and emotional bandwidth, current circumstances being what they were, to stick to the program, which would require me to weigh and measure portions of food, write everything down in the tracker, come to weekly meetings, clean junk food out of the cupboards, calculate point values for the food that remained, and exercise on a regular basis. But I needed the boundaries and control the program offered.

"Hi there," the familiar-looking woman behind the counter said when it was my turn to weigh in.

I handed her a clipboard with the new/rejoining member paperwork I'd completed, dropped my purse onto a nearby chair, and kicked off my sneakers.

"Ready when you are," she said.

I'm never ready. "Great!"

Here I was again, about to step on a scale and judge my worth.

Thirty-three years. For thirty-three years, I'd gone through periods of weighing myself daily, sometimes twice daily, morning and night—and, in high school, I'd weighed in at some Weight Watchers meetings too. In college, I brought a scale to the dorm and weighed myself in my room. I weighed myself during my semester abroad on my French family's scale, converting kilos to pounds with a calculator. Later, I weighed myself in gyms and at personalized meetings with one-on-one consultants at Jenny Craig and Lindora. I weighed myself in secret in friends' and family members' homes, before and after wedding dress fittings, and mere days after giving birth. The numbers had tracked my journey inching toward or skyrocketing away from feeling acceptable. Here I was, again.

The receptionist was waiting. I took a breath, stepped onto the pad, the digital readout blinking red. I willed the number to be lower than I expected. It caught: 196.

Fuck.

"Got it," the woman said, expressionless.

I stepped off the scale. *Cow.*

She affixed the sticker in my booklet, handed it back. I scooped up my belongings, plopped into one of the few remaining seats toward the back, pulled my shoes on. *How could you let yourself get so far gone?*

I cut myself no slack, ashamed of my too big body and lack of willpower. My lowest adult weight, the number I'd hit back when I was coming here and seeing Dolly for therapy, had been 152. Not great, but not awful. As the years had marched forward, the pounds had crept back on, into the low 170s—the same twenty pounds I'd been duking it out with for forever. Today's weight, 196, was only seven pounds shy of a few days after I gave birth. One hundred ninety-six pounds was a man's weight, and more than Theo weighed on our wedding day. Theo had never minded my weight, called me his beautiful bride then and now. He'd always loved my hourglass shape—thinner waist, larger hips—regardless of what the scale said. But for me, 196 pounds represented failure.

Dolly called the meeting to order.

She would have followed the normal routine, starting with awards: red bookmarks imprinted with the words *I LOST 5 POUNDS* for people who'd lost their first five pounds, star stickers printed with a 5 for anyone who'd lost additional weight in five-pound increments to affix to said bookmark, blue bookmarks that read *I LOST 25 POUNDS* for anyone who had, and key chains to anyone who'd lost ten percent of their weight.

In between, we would have dutifully clapped—the positive reinforcement a must. Dolly would have reminded anyone who was new to stay after the meeting for a review of how the Weight Watchers points system worked, and she would have announced the week's Weight Watchers–approved topic.

Whatever it was, something like tips and tricks for eating out or tips and tricks for portion control or tips and tricks to make exercise enjoyable, she would have glossed over it to focus instead on something she found more important, like the impact of shame on eating habits. She would have opened a discussion, and someone would probably have cried.

It could have been me.

HOME

Chili simmered in the Crock-Pot. Cornbread cooled on the counter. Faith had requested this meal for her welcome home dinner. Six days after Dr. Amanda had sent her to the hospital, I'd spent the morning keeping my nerves in check by chopping, stirring, browning, measuring, and simmering. Now, I was glued to the kitchen window, waiting for Theo's Buick to glide by.

The car hit my sight line, and I bolted to the foot of the driveway. Through the passenger window, I could see Faith's profile. I searched her features for any clue as to how she was feeling, but one eye and half a mouth told me nothing. She got out, wearing her own jeans and a frown. *Uh-oh*. "Welcome home, ba—"

"I feel exactly the same as when I left," she said, bursting into tears. She thrust herself into my arms, her forehead digging into my shoulder. "I'm not any better, and I gained *ten* fucking pounds."

Persistent hunger was a side effect of the antidepressant medication, and Faith hadn't been allowed to know her weight since treatment began, back with Mona. Knowing she'd gained a few pounds meant they'd weighed her at the hospital—another breach in eating disorder protocol.

"Okay, sweetheart," I said, rubbing her back. I watched Theo close the driver-side door. I could tell by the tight look on his face that the ride home had stressed him out. Across the street, I noticed how tall the neighbor's palm trees had grown. Giant plumes of spiky green fronds sitting atop their nubby trunks obscured our view of Boney Peak. We'd have to mention that. "Let's get inside and try to relax." It was far too soon to think bringing her home was a mistake.

At the door, the aroma of warm cumin and spicy chili powder wafted toward us.

"Mmm, that smells good," Faith said, teary-eyed.

"Good. I made the cornbread you asked for too."

Inside, she sank to the living room floor to pet the cat. Theo banged through the front door with Faith's suitcase. "Where do you want her stuff?"

"Her room. I'll take care of it later."

Theo headed down the hallway. Faith followed him and I followed her, tense.

In the doorway, Faith stopped short. "Where's my stuff?"

My hand floated to my throat. "The spare room," I said. "We wanted to help you stay safe."

"We can put everything back up with duct tape," Theo rushed to add. "And we thought you might be ready for that bedroom makeover."

"I guess," Faith said, looking crestfallen.

The three of us stood, silent. The absence of posters, dream catcher, corkboard, and bric-a-brac highlighted the childish nature of Noah and his many arks. The heap of stuffed animals overflowed out of the hot-pink plastic baby doll crib.

Faith noticed the fresh flowers I'd placed on her dresser. Her favorites: colorful pink, yellow, and orange Gerbera daisies. The first hint of a smile.

That evening, when we got our food, I didn't portion out my chili with a measuring cup. The very last thing Faith needed to know was that I was trying to diet, again, while she struggled with an eating disorder. So I plopped approximately a cup's worth into my bowl, sprinkled on a small amount of grated cheddar cheese, eschewed the sour cream, and cut a small piece of cornbread. No dessert.

The two or three days immediately following Faith's return were chock-full of errands, doing everything I could think of to keep our bodies—and, hopefully, our brains—busy.

Faith's friends were in school, so the two of us went to a movie. We picked up some new art supplies. She still loved to draw, color, and paint. We bought a few new clothing items for her and went for a hike. As I huffed and puffed, she literally ran circles around me, exuberant to be in nature.

I purchased a membership for Faith at the local YMCA, and took her for an overdue orthodontist appointment. Theo focused on the bedroom makeover. He took Faith to Home Depot for paint (eggplant) and taught her how to strip wallpaper. Music and laughter (naughty *The Book of Mormon*!) returned to the house. I prepared simple meals, and we ate them. She didn't run off to purge or lock herself in the bathroom—a sense of fragile normalcy.

Faith met her new therapist. Together, they negotiated with me that Faith should be allowed fifteen minutes of alone time at home in her room whenever she felt overwhelmed and needed a break. I shared that news with Theo, whose forehead creased. "I know," I said. But the therapist came highly recommended by Kim, and we so badly wanted our plan to work. He'd purchased a fire-engine-red Craftsman toolbox into which we'd locked the kitchen knives, scissors, pizza cutter, and vegetable peelers. Every foreseeable variable was accounted for, and Faith had signed a safety contract at the hospital prior to coming home.

We all tried our hardest to cooperate and follow instructions. We did. But then, Theo and I were still Theo and I. Faith was still Faith. Each day since Faith had gotten home, her anxiety was escalating. I tried to look at it from her point of view. She'd been thrust at one stranger after another, then more strangers, one new environment after another. Sent away entirely. Hospitalized. Everyone telling her that what she was doing was wrong, dangerous. To take responsibility for herself. What did that even mean?

ROCK BOTTOM

It's the unforeseeable variable that gets you. I'd overlooked the framed pictures on Faith's dresser. Each one covered with a thin piece of glass.

911. Police. Paramedics. Gurney. Ambulance. No trying to convince anyone to let our daughter remain at home. My plan had failed, and I knew it. Theo spoke to the officer and handed my purse to me as I followed the gurney. "I'll follow you in the car," he said.

Thirty minutes later, Faith and I were inside a cubicle in the emergency room at our local hospital. Theo hadn't yet arrived.

"What's going on?" asked the nurse.

"I want to hurt myself," Faith said, prostrate on a hospital bed.

Next to her, I rocked from side to side, as if in a trance, the glare of the fluorescent lights striking me from every glossy surface. I was trying to come to grips with this development, what it meant. The nurse, a stethoscope slung around her neck, scurried about her work. The pain of failure spilled out of my head and down my spine, branching out to every other part of me with the single, relentless demand to FIX THIS. Pressure made my hands and feet tingle. Ready for action. But there was nothing I could do. A digital clock, mounted on the wall, big red numbers, counted up as the seconds ticked by.

The nurse told me to step out so Faith could change. Theo arrived and while Faith was still with the nurse, the two of us waited, lost in thought, until the nurse finally called us in.

Faith's clothes were folded on the counter, and she wore a hospital gown and a light blanket. She looked young and pale and small. "Are you guys angry?" she asked.

"No," Theo and I said in unison.

"I'm sorry."

"We're not mad, angel," I said, grabbing her hand.

"You have nothing to be sorry about," Theo added.

"Let's see what we've got here," the nurse said, exposing Faith's thigh.

I whimpered. Theo let out a long, loud breath.

"The doctor's going to need to take a look at these," the nurse said. "I'll be back. One of you needs to stay in here at all times."

The three of us settled down to wait out the long night ahead. Eventually, a doctor would arrive to attend the wounds, as would a representative from the children's response team to tell us what we already knew: Faith would be on another psychiatric hold. A nurse would tell us that because our local hospital didn't have a psychiatric department and there was no open bed at ones that did, we'd have to wait. However long it took.

There was a process. A procedure. We sat. We waited. We waited some more. I'd run out the door with my purse, but hadn't had time to grab my book. I was too tired to read, anyway.

A couple of hours later, Faith asked what time it was.

"Just after nine," I said.

"You have to tell me when it's midnight so we can sing 'Happy Birthday' to Dad."

Theo shook his head. "It's okay, baby doll."

"No, I want to," she said.

Three hours later, at midnight, when the clock with the big red numbers read 00:00:00, Faith and I sang "Happy Birthday" to Theo. He smiled as best he could, crossing and recrossing his legs.

"Why don't you head home," I said to him. "It doesn't make any sense for both of us to sit here all night. Go get some sleep."

I closed the door then, pulling the curtain shut too, and turning down the lights, grateful for our cocoon, insulated against the ER's late-night chaos.

"This is all my fault," Faith said, toying with the thin blanket. "I'm sorry, Mom, and now I've ruined Dad's birthday."

I didn't know how to comfort her beyond saying what I'd said the last time she took the blame. "None of this is anyone's fault, love." I was actually beginning to believe it about myself too. Sort of. "Try to get some rest."

Faith drifted off to sleep, and I tried to get comfortable on the thinly padded wooden chair using the bed as a pillow, but no position worked.

"Move over a little, babe," I whispered. We settled into a spoon, just like we had on the long-ago night when I'd noticed her first scratch, just like we had on so many, many nights before and after.

Through the thin mattress, metal dug into pressure points: my ankle, thigh, hip, shoulder. I draped my free arm over Faith, careful to avoid the wounded area. My other arm, pinned beneath me, tingled. Next, my ear. I tried to ignore the discomfort, sinking instead into the feeling of Faith snug against my body. The back of her head, her hair, was inches from my face. I smelled her familiar airy scent tinged with bleach.

Everywhere around us, boxes of this, vials of that, equipment. Every available inch of space designed and utilized for the sole purpose of saving lives, relieving physical pain. Above and beside us, in wards, on units, and in surgeries, sick people, hurt people, damaged people lived or died. Ours was a different kind of emergency. Lying in the dim coolness, I longed to drift off into blissful sleep, but my churning thoughts said no.

My daughter had become a girl whose future I could no longer discern. Worse, feared. I imagined a revolving door of first responders, hospital stays, white coats, and failed treatments. Would that be it for us?

My world was on this gurney. Nothing else mattered. This moment, right now, was all there was. Faith, safe in my arms, was enough. It had to be.

TRANSITIONS

Nineteen hours. That's how long we waited in the local emergency room for a bed on an adolescent psychiatric ward to open. Nineteen long, sad, boring, and frustrating hours.

I didn't argue with Faith after she asked for and then refused the muffin I walked the full length of the hospital to buy. But I ate it not long after I ate mine, officially ditching my diet until some future point in time. I didn't argue when Theo put news on the television. I didn't roll my eyes when the technician arrived to draw Faith's blood but had no idea why it needed to be tested. And I didn't tell the parade of disembodied heads, peeking into our cubicle to say there was no update on an available bed, this whole situation was a crock of shit. I simply sat, in acceptance, still wearing the prior day's clothes, yearning for my toothbrush—an odd sense of relief, my thoughts not bouncing between the past and the future. I was just there, in the moment.

A bed finally opened up thirty miles away in Ventura. A flurry of activity. Protocol dictated that Faith be transported via ambulance, and, oddly, the same two EMTs who'd ferried us to the ER reappeared to strap Faith to a stretcher and roll her out the automated door. I followed. Theo ran for the car.

The next day, Faith was safely ensconced on the adolescent ward at Aurora Vista del Mar. I wandered around the house, resigned. I stood at the threshold of her room looking at her unused bed, unused book bag, unused notepads. I'd never consciously thought about the expectations I'd had for Faith. But now, because they'd come into question, I acknowledged them: school, career, marriage, family. Normal. Ordinary. The same ones my parents had had for me. But illness had thrown my fantasies for a loop.

Fantasy versus reality. The discrepancy hurt. *Whose fault is that?* Not Faith's. The only expectation that seemed fair to have was none. And not because of illness. I wanted Faith to choose her life's path, not follow one out of obligation. For her sake and mine, I would try to take each day at face value. No more, no less.

Later, Theo and I drove to Ventura for visiting hours. The only difference between this hospital stay and the first one was Faith's comfort level. She seemed the first couple of days to almost enjoy herself, to feel at home and accepted among her struggling peers. That idea scared the hell out of me. Before we could have a formal conversation as to the length of her stay, she got upset about something, tried to reopen her healing wounds, and the decision was taken out of our hands, again. She'd stay until the next step was resolved, which would be a new residential treatment facility.

I found The AG Center, located in LA's Koreatown neighborhood. Prior to committing, skittish over our experience with the first place, Theo and I visited the site. Another converted house in another nondescript, sprawling part of downtown. We met the staff, told our story. I shared our fears about the way Faith had been kicked out of LV by the powers that be, wondering aloud what a repeat of that experience might do to us. Therapists and administrators explained their twelve-steppy philosophy and, like the first place, focus on regimentation and behavior modification. No other model seemed to exist. But the admin in charge allayed our concerns by pledging to never give up on our fourteen-year-old daughter. We formulated a plan for Faith to be transferred the following week from the hospital to AG.

BATTLE ARMOR, KIT REPACK

Dumped, sorted, verified, restored:
Wallet
Cash
Tchotchkes
Compact
Pen
Cell phone
Tissues
Photo keeper
Checkbook
Notepad
Band-Aids
ChapStick
Cough drops
Lotion
Eye drops
Treatment document
Granola bars
Cutting, by Steven Levenkron

THE WHOLE PERSON WHEEL

Twenty days after Faith arrived at The AG Center, our seventeenth wedding anniversary. It was April 20, a Saturday—mandatory parent participation for family group therapy. Structured exercises, discussion of therapeutic materials and how to use them to improve our familial relationships—not what I'd ever expected to be doing on an anniversary, but I was happy the three of us were together.

On this particular day, in the house's living room, Faith sat to my left. Theo to my right. We'd received the assignment and a small pile of heavily trafficked crayons. One paper—"The Whole Person Wheel"—had a pie chart divided into six equal slices, individually labeled with the words *physical*, *emotional*, *volitional*, *social*, *mental*, and *spiritual*. Another sheet explained the Whole Person Model, proposing that human beings embody these six potentials, or basic needs, all of which require attention for a person to be happy. The Whole Person Model said I should think of a person as a wheel: damage one part, and the whole thing stops rolling. That made sense to me. In graduate school, I'd gravitated toward family systems theory, which sees a family less as a collection of individuals and more as an interconnected system. If one person hurt, the whole hurt. If one person healed, the whole healed a little too. At least, I sure hoped so.

Our task today was to rate how well we were meeting each of the six basic needs categories on a scale of zero to one hundred percent. If we'd fulfilled, say, fifty percent of our *spiritual* need, we would color half the slice. Self-worth, the worksheet said, is the result of all six needs being met. *This oughta be interesting.*

To my right, Theo was coloring away. To my left, Faith was penning a picture on the back of one of her papers, a girl who looked a lot like her. Tears dripped down picture girl's cheeks; a gaping hole in her chest exposed a heart encased by spiderwebs. Her pen scratched against the tabletop. *Scratch, scratch, scratch.* The sound pierced my eardrums. Faith hadn't cut since she'd arrived at AG. They were keeping a closer eye than the last place, but progress with the eating disorder, depression, and anxiety was going slowly.

I stared at my blank pie chart. How could I accurately rate my fulfillment of these needs? I was tempted to lie and just color in a majority of every slice. Why not? But then I pictured myself, three days earlier, sitting next to Theo in our local high school auditorium. Incoming freshman orientation day. We couldn't know what would happen next with Faith's education, but we'd shown up for the meeting anyway. Around us, a sea of smiling moms and dads. People chatting. The atmosphere light, congenial. I'd avoided making eye contact, in case any of Faith's friends' parents were there. Questions would have required answers. A woman had taken the microphone, introduced herself as the principal, and explained the transition from middle school. More smiles. A mom's head leaning on a dad's shoulder. And then the principal had said, "If your kid graduates from this high school and wants to go to college, they'll get in. It's just that simple."

Faith flipped her paper over to start the assignment, and I, too, hunkered down with my crayons.

Among the six needs, *physical* seemed easiest to assess. I considered my thick brown hair, hazel eyes, button nose. My freckles, which reminded me of Dad, my Irish heritage. Then I thought of my chubby cheeks, droopy chin, rounded stomach, hips, and thighs. But my health was good! No weight-related health issues like diabetes, high blood pressure, or high cholesterol. I exercised, sometimes. Was there a middle ground? Maybe sixty percent? My gut said no, too low. Okay, good. Seventy percent? Hell no. Way too high. *Split the difference.* With the purple crayon, still my favorite color, I colored in approximately sixty-five percent of the physical slice.

I completed the five remaining needs—*emotional*, *volitional*, *social*, *mental*, *spiritual*—in the same way as the first. Think. Color. Think. Color. Finally, I set my crayons down to assess. I'd only filled in about a third of my *spiritual* and *emotional* wedges. The rest were higher, but still. So much white space.

On the table in front of me, piles of broken crayons and shredded wrappers. They smelled like dirt and chemicals. Faith was drawing purple stars around her pie chart. Sideways, in big purple letters, she'd written the words "Kill the Worthless." I vaguely sensed this phrase was from a heavy metal song, but I couldn't be sure.

"Okay," said Joel, the primary therapist. "I'd like us to go around the room, and you'll each read your numbers out loud and tell us why you chose what you chose."

Damn it. If I had known we'd be sharing, I'd have gone ahead and inflated my numbers after all! My palms itched, and I rubbed them against my pants.

"Who wants to go first?" Joel asked.

Silence. Everyone fidgeted. I had always been a *teacher, teacher, pick me* sort, but those days were long over. People looked up, down, all around.

"I'll go," one of the moms finally said, breaking the tension.

Every parent's and even every kid's numbers looked pretty much alike: almost everyone had rated themselves high—eighties, nineties, even one hundred percent—in almost every category. Sure, most people, especially the kids, had picked one area that needed attention and was less robustly colored—and Joel asked everyone what they could do to improve on their lowest rating.

My blood pounded in my ears and I began to sweat. I was an outlier.

"Okay, Yokas family," Joel said. "You're up."

"I'll go," Theo said.

He talked numbers, reasoning. I glanced at his paper and saw that his answers mirrored the group's. I was unsurprised. Self-assurance had attracted me to him from the start. When he got to the *volitional* need, about exerting our will, not our willpower, and accepting what we cannot change, he quoted the serenity prayer. Then, about the *mental* need, he said, "It's one hundred percent, due to the clarity of my cognition."

Okayyyyy. In Theo's opinion, clarity of cognition resulted from only one factor: sobriety. His biggest problem, he said, was the *emotional* category—our ability to deal with our own and other people's feelings in healthy ways. Only twenty percent fulfillment. His dad had taught him that emotions were a sign of weakness, but he knew it wasn't true.

Huh. That comment hit the mark.

"How can you improve on it?" Joel asked.

"I have to believe all this therapy will help me get better at dealing with my emotions," Theo said. "Tracey's and Faith's too."

That answer irked me. No action plan, no pledge to change anything. But it wasn't my place in this setting to say so. Now Joel was looking at me.

I looked at my chart, opened my mouth.

Everyone in the room stared at me with bionic eyes that bored through my skull into my brain. I felt trapped. My throat clamped shut. My head burnt with shame and felt like it weighed one hundred pounds, my inadequacies taking on actual weight and mass and volume. What the fuck was wrong with me?

Seconds ticked by.

You have to speak!

Nothing.

Just say something. Anything.

I stared at all the white space on my chart. No way in hell would I speak my numbers out loud. "I'm not going to read them all," I said, my cheeks burning hot. Joel opened his mouth, but I plowed on. "I'll talk about spirituality. Thirty percent. That's the one I want to work on the most. It's something the three of us are interested in, in our own ways, and it's something I can explore myself and we can explore as a family. I was raised Catholic and feel like I'm still trying to recover."

"Okay," Joel butted in. "And it's important to remember that we're not necessarily talking about religion."

"Correct," I said.

"What can you do?" Joel asked.

"I'm working on it, reading books, exploring alternatives. That's all I have to say." I crossed my arms, fixed my gaze on my chart. So much white space.

I was transfixed by the physical manifestation, on a flimsy sheet of printer paper, of my low self-esteem. No amount of pretending I was someone else had changed the fundamental truth, and the effort to keep myself together made me tremble.

Once before, during a grad school family tree exercise, I'd had a visceral reaction to seeing my life on a piece of paper. The point then was to use form and symbol to visualize patterns and factors like ill health, divorce, addiction, premature death, and suicide permeating our family structure. I'd cried handing it to the teacher. But that sadness paled in comparison to now.

Joel turned to Faith. She leaned over her paper, which was

lying flat on the table, and jumped right in. "Like my mom was saying, about religion and stuff. I'm kinda confused about all that. I listed spirituality as twenty percent. That's pretty low." Her physical, she said, was half of one percent. "Because, ya know, I have an eating disorder and pretty much hate my body." A breezy tone contrasted with the cruel words, and in the *physical* slice, a miniscule brown dot, smaller than the size of a pea. *Wrong.*

Anyone who can swim laps for an hour straight should not pick half of one percent fulfillment of *physical* need. If we were there for any reason besides mental illness, I might have laughed out loud. My eyes slid back and forth between our charts. Her color scheme, albeit limited to the ones we'd been given, was so dark. Purple, yes, and a splash of red in the *mental* slice. But predominantly black and brown. None of the yellow, orange, blue, and green featured in Theo's and mine.

"My social's thirty percent," she continued, "because I don't have friends." *Wrong again.*

She had lots of friends at home, had already made friends in treatment. As Faith spoke, her shoulder-length hair hung down, hiding her face. The body she'd just maligned curled inward, as if her very cells were recoiling from the disdain.

Faith explained her confusion around the *emotional* slice; because she was so "emo" and "couldn't deal," she'd changed her high number to a lower one. Indeed, she'd scribbled out half of what she'd colored in. Again, my eyes slid between our charts. She'd colored as carefully inside the lines as I had, but where I'd colored my slices in the shape of slices, Faith had kept her colors more centered, in a shape that resembled a wonky hexagon.

What glared up at me from the tabletop was not the color or the shape, not how neat or messy, but the white space. Far more white space even than mine.

The person I loved most in the world thought even less of herself than I thought of myself.

For nine long months, I'd been struggling to accept that Faith's illness was not my fault. Professionals had told me so. We'd discussed nature versus nurture, my mother's death, and the fact that mental illness was one of life's difficult realities. But looking at Faith's chart, I could not shake the idea that, but for me and my bloodlines, we would not be here. We would not be sitting in treatment and Faith would know how to love herself.

1981

I stood in front of my closet, trying to decide what to wear the next day for the start of eighth grade. Puppy and kitten posters from Scholastic, along with a few pullout pictures from *Tiger Beat* magazine of Shaun Cassidy, Scott Baio, and Lance Kerwin lined the walls. My *Star Wars* record blasted, but not too loud. I could, when I felt like it, recite the entire album's worth of dialogue. *Help me, Obi-Wan Kenobi. You're my only hope.* God, I'd give anything to be Princess Leia, gallivanting across the galaxy with Luke, Han, and Chewie. Instead, I had to try on clothes.

I flicked through hangers. Mom had been bugging me about going shopping, but I was thirteen years old now. Had better things to do than be seen at the mall with my mommy, and when I told her I wanted a pair of Calvin Kleins, like Brooke Shields, she'd said, "I refuse to spend that kind of money on a pair of pants." Dad still wasn't working a regular job after his heart surgery, so we were always arguing about how much stuff cost. I couldn't wait to grow up, get a job, and buy whatever the hell I wanted.

I pulled a pair of boring, regular jeans out of the closet, imagined the look on Mom's face when Scott Baio rang the doorbell. *Tiger Beat* was always hosting a contest: Enter to win a meet and greet! I always entered. I could get teary-eyed just thinking about Scott or Shaun or anyone whisking me away to Hollywood.

A lightsaber's *shrumm mmmm* sound burst out of the speaker.

I dropped my terry-cloth shorts—the ones I'd spent all summer in—and stepped into the jeans. I pulled them up. But uh-oh. They got stuck at my hips. Shit. I threw them on the floor. Next!

"Come on," I said, wiggling and waggling. Bumpy looked at me like I was an oddball. Nope. This pair didn't fit either. I was running out of options fast.

The corduroys? Those I could get up, but the zipper wouldn't close, even when I sucked in my belly. I grabbed the last pair from the closet and Nestea-plunged onto my bed. I tugged the button side toward the hole side, but I couldn't close the divide.

I sat up, pant front splayed open like a V, belly bulging into the gap. Nothing fit. *Fat ass*. Needless to say, Dr. Emma's diet had been a spectacular failure. It wasn't her fault. I just couldn't keep my mouth shut, and Mom had quit bugging me about eating a long time ago.

The mall was already closed. What was I going to do? Suddenly, Luke, Leia, and Han were getting on my nerves, and I turned the volume down. I needed to think.

Dad. He might have a suggestion. I walked across the hall. He was laid out on the bed, reading. "Dad." I hesitated. Light glinted off the brass headboard. He put his book down. "What can I do you for?" he asked.

I felt ashamed, like a loser. I didn't want to admit the truth, but I didn't know what else to do. For sure, I wasn't going to tell Mom. I took a breath. "None of my pants fit."

"Oh. Okay. Try a pair of mine," he said, without missing a beat.

His? "Um. Which ones?"

"Jeans, that drawer," he answered, pointing. If he was upset about me needing a larger size, he didn't say anything. He wanted to help me.

In my bedroom, I tried on Dad's pants. He'd lost weight after the heart surgery, I reasoned, so while they were too big, it was nothing one of his belts and an oversize T-shirt couldn't hide. I looked at myself in the mirror, wishing I could disappear.

"They work?" Dad called out.

"They're fine," I said, closing the door. I took Dad's pants off, put my shorts back on. I turned the sound back up on my record player, opened my sketchbook, and grabbed a pencil. I kept trying to get the exact right shape for R2-D2. My thoughts floated away to the future, when everything would be better, to fantasies of romance and adventure in outer space.

PART THREE

1992

The bar was packed, the DJ spinning upbeat tunes, lights flashing, bartenders mixing strong drinks. Perfect. But one sure way to feel invisible—being the fat chick in a bar. Alcohol reduced my inhibitions, made me feel sexy. And drinking made it easier to believe guys saw me that way too.

I'd turned twenty-four years old two weeks prior, and my friend, Collette, who I'd met at a temp job—two college-educated women making copies eight hours a day and stapling them together—had invited me out this evening to celebrate my birthday. And my new job. First big promotion in the entertainment biz: from gofer to production coordinator on *The Jerry Lewis Telethon*. Soon, I'd be leaving for a month on location in Las Vegas. I couldn't wait to prove to my boss what I could do.

Handing me a drink, Collette yelled over the music, "Are you excited?"

"Can't fucking wait," I yelled back. "Thanks!" I held up my glass. We clinked.

My drink, probably a sweet sloe-gin fizz, went down easy. And fast.

We chatted and drank, drank and chatted. Music pounded. Lights flashed. A while later, a couple of single guys from over at the bar worked their way toward us. They put shots on the table.

"Whooo-hoooo," I cheered, gulping.

We called the waitress over, ordered a few more shots.

The DJ lowered the music, got our attention. "Any woman out there tonight willing to remove her bra?" Who knew what had prompted that. Weird shit happened all the time in bars.

Oh, my god. Yes! I was wearing a strapless! I raised my hand. "Me!" I yelled. "Me!"

Collette was laughing. The guys cheered me on.

"Come on then," the DJ said into the microphone. "Let's see it!"

I reached under my shirt, swiped off my bra, and twirled it over my head, like Wonder Woman with her lasso. We were rewarded with a few more shots.

My eyelids fluttered open. I blinked a couple of times. Seated, on a floor. Bathroom stall door. My cheek was resting on the toilet seat. Oh god. I must have passed out. I was still in the bar. Good. I couldn't have been in there too long; someone would have found me.

Shaking, I stood up. My head was pounding, but I made my way to the sink, splashed water on my face. I studied my reflection: flat hair, mascara-rimmed eyes, puffy cheeks. What the fuck was wrong with me? At least I wasn't in some guy's bed.

I grabbed paper towels, blotted my face. I had to get out of there, had to work in the morning and couldn't be late. I had the only key to the production office. *You need to get a grip on yourself.*

I stepped into the bar, stopped short. It was empty. Dark. *What the . . . ?*

It had closed for the night with me still in the bathroom. The bathroom was next to the front door. I yanked. It didn't budge.

"Oh, shit," I said out loud. This was before cell phones. "Hello?" I hoped someone was still here somewhere. No answer. I was afraid to move, feared setting off an alarm. That's when I noticed the pay phone. What choice did I have?

"911, what is your emergency?" the operator said.

"Uh, I fell asleep and now I'm locked inside a bar and can't get out," I said, humiliated. I prided myself on never needing help.

"You mean you passed out?" she said, snarky.

Rude. I didn't know why that mattered. "Yeah, but I need to get out of here."

"I'll send a unit."

A few minutes later, eyes peered in through the front door glass. "You're definitely stuck," the officer said, holding up a chain and padlock.

"Can you call someone?" I asked.

"Like who? Were you here alone?"

I told him about my friend.

"Get her over here," he ordered.

I called her collect.

Just then, a security guard from the mall next door putted up in his golf cart to say there was a door at the back of the bar that opened from the inside. By the time I walked around to the front, Collette had arrived. She looked as bad as I felt. The cop was reading her the riot act for leaving me behind.

I probably shouldn't have been driving yet, but I got in my car, headed home. Replaying the evening over and over in my mind, I chortled. It was the sound of recognition, the sound of consequences escaped. I shook my head, turned up the radio. Images invaded my mind: jail cell, violent attack, bloody outcome, worse. *Damn it, stop.* I turned the radio up louder. Hit the gas pedal harder. Anything to shut down the loop playing in my mind.

OJAI

I unpacked the few toiletries Theo and I had brought to the resort for our anniversary celebration. Stored my bulging purse, which contained our pie charts, in the closet, where I planned to leave it for the remainder of the weekend—out of sight, out of mind. Three hours earlier, at the end of the whole person wheel session, we'd hugged Faith goodbye. She'd told us to have fun, and I could tell she'd meant it. Theo and I deserved this respite, but I still felt guilty on a getaway with Faith in treatment.

Theo was on the phone confirming his tee time for the morning. I grabbed my book, walked to the balcony, and sank into a chaise. Beyond the railing, a golf course. Lush fairways stretched toward distant silvery mountains. Rosebushes plump with white, pink, and coral flowers extended left and right. Foliage, verdant and leafy, in colors ranging from sage to fern to moss. The lavishness hurt my eyes and soothed my soul.

Uninvited images of broken crayons and tiny brown dots invaded my mind. My heart started pounding, again. As incredible as it sounds, only now was I realizing how drastically I had underestimated what Faith's healing would entail. I was about to fall into the rabbit hole of perseveration. *No*. This was our anniversary.

I focused on my book, *Seeking Peace*, by Mary Pipher, chosen specifically for its subtitle: *Chronicles of the Worst Buddhist in the World*. I'd done spotty investigation into Buddhism, gravitated toward its principle regarding suffering—that suffering exists, there is a cause for it, and there can be an end to it. I certainly wanted to learn how to suffer less, and I wanted to help Faith suffer less too.

Theo hung up. "All set?" I asked.

"All set," he said. "I'm gonna change."

I opened *Seeking Peace* to the dog-eared page. "I made another important decision," Pipher, a well-known therapist, wrote. "I was finished with the self-improvement projects I had launched my whole life. All of my goals to better myself had become gaols, prisons that kept me from accepting myself. My constant efforts to improve had been a form of self-aggression." I put the book back down. *Seriously?* I thought, again. Same as the first time I'd read those words.

My pie chart clearly demonstrated the need for a massive self-improvement project. Could Pipher be saying that the way to better oneself is to not have the goal to better oneself?

It was definitely time for a glass of wine.

In the restaurant, the maître d' seated Theo and me at a table next to a large picture window. A waiter swooped in with two flutes of champagne. "Compliments of the house," he said.

"Oh, thank you," I beamed. I'd indicated while making the reservation that we were celebrating an anniversary.

Theo ordered iced tea, but I didn't wait. "Happy anniversary, dear," I said, clinking his water glass. The cool liquid hit my lips, and bubbles tickled my nose.

"Enjoy it," he said. "I really want you to relax."

His ulterior motive: sex, of course.

Theo's frustration had increased to the point that he'd questioned whether we'd have sex ever again, and he'd recently demanded to know if I'd gone out and found a boyfriend. At that, I'd laughed out loud.

Even if I had been interested in sex, which I clearly was not, when would I have had time to find a boyfriend? And what guy was going to be interested in an overweight, middle-aged, married woman consumed with her daughter's illness? As the months had ticked by, I'd retreated further and further into myself until my softer side had disappeared. But sitting in this sanctuary, it was our anniversary. Time to reconnect, to put our relationship first.

Theo looked at me over a flickering candle. "You look pretty tonight."

I was wearing a dress. "Thanks. So do you." Clean-shaven, trimmed eyebrows. "I love that shirt." Hawaiian—cheerful palm trees, colorful surfboards.

"I love you, you know," he said. "Forever and a day." The words we'd had engraved on our wedding bands.

"Forever and a day," I said.

I still didn't feel invested in putting our marriage ahead of my mothering duties and responsibilities, and I knew how unfair that was to Theo. This night in particular, hours after completing that deplorable whole person assignment, I felt tender and entitled. I wanted to dissolve into sleep-induced oblivion, but we deserved a celebration. I switched my empty flute for his full one.

I looked out the window. "Oh! It's starting," I said.

Dusk, the sun's rays hitting the mountain, reflected a pink hue from the sky to the ground. Ojai is known for the "pink moment." It looked like a shower of pastel rain. Beyond the glass, greens looked greener, reds redder, browns inviting. Nature in soft focus, the antithesis of treatment and hospital settings. A feeling of awe crept into my chest, something I hadn't felt in a long time. My whole body relaxed. Minutes later, the sun set low enough for the show to end.

"Wow," I said.

We ate—braised short ribs for two with a nice cabernet for me. The meat flaked off the bone. Savory herbs and spices. We chatted, avoiding topics like damaged wheels, chaotic emotions, and mental illness. We wiped our plates clean with crusts of bread. Dessert arrived with a lit sparkler and the words "Happy Anniversary" written in chocolate sauce around the plate's edge. We ate that too.

Back in our room, Theo wasted no time stripping naked and hopping into bed. He clicked through TV channels looking for music. Knowing his expectation for the evening, I'd packed a crumpled, decade-old teddy I'd found in a ball at the bottom of my pajama drawer. I grabbed it now, sidestepping into the bathroom.

Alcohol and sugar had done their job. The relentless ache that existed deep in my core had dulled. I felt sated and loved. Pie charts, under- and over-inflated numbers, and self-improvement projects were nowhere on my radar. I stripped off my dress, slid the teddy over my head. Full-length mirror on the bathroom door. Ugh.

Far too tight, the teddy highlighted every bump, curve, and bulge. But I knew Theo wouldn't care, and I resisted an urge to wrap myself in one of the luxurious hotel robes.

"I love your outfit," Theo said, tossing back the covers.

"I figured you would."

I snuggled next to him. He kissed me and I kissed him back. "Thanks for the close shave," I said, looking into his warm brown eyes.

"No chafing allowed," he joked. "Besides, you're so gorgeous I have to keep up. You haven't changed a bit in seventeen years."

I bark-laughed. "I don't know about that."

"I do."

Theo slid his hand up my leg to my hip. Calluses snagged the teddy's lacy material. He traced the ridgeline of my hip into the dip at my waist. "I love this part," he said, reaching for the light switch. "You're still my beautiful bride."

BILL OF GOODS

"That candle smells good," I said, sitting across from Kim for my weekly session.

It was Monday, two days after the pie chart. I'd successfully avoided thinking about my damaged wheel long enough to eat dinner and have sex, but the respite had ended the following morning and I'd been thinking a jumbled negative mess ever since.

"How was the getaway?" she asked.

"Fine," I said, bursting into tears. Damn, I was sick and tired of crying. I blew my nose, explained the whole person assignment, my chart, Faith's chart, everyone else's high numbers, and my refusal to say all of mine. "I can only imagine what those people thought of me. We've been talking for months about my guilt and inadequacy. Why can't I let go of feeling responsible?"

"We have to move into some more shame work."

"Got plenty of that," I sighed. "I feel like a failure, and now I have proof I was right."

Kim cocked her head. A sure sign she was about to challenge me. "That's a lot to get from one piece of paper."

"Maybe, but it's true."

"Okay. So what's your takeaway?"

"It's the opposite of what we're taught," I said.

"How so?"

I leaned in. "Right from the start we're taught to take care of everyone else's needs before our own, to prioritize others. We're selfish if we don't. That's what I learned anyway, that I was selfish. And it's even more true for mothers. A good mother puts her child's needs, her family's needs, ahead of her own. We're a disappointment if we say no. I think I'm seeing with this chart that the system is backward." I stopped, frustrated, searching for more words. "I guess what I'm trying to say is, the whole point of taking care of myself is to live the healthier behavior I hope for, for the people I love. Do instead of say." I leaned back.

Mom came to mind. The way we'd argued when I was a kid about any number of things, her incessant smoking being near the top of the list. She had never cared how I felt about the stink of the smoke, the ash getting everywhere, including up my nose, or that I'd begged her to stop. And sometime back then, we'd learned that secondhand smoke can kill. When she'd deigned to respond, she'd launch into a story about herself and end, inexplicably, with a directive for me not to become a smoker. "Hypocrite," I'd say. "Do as I say, not as I do," she would say, and about more than just smoking. The message being, *I'll do whatever I want, and you should do what I want too.* What kind of message was that?

But I realized I'd repeated a similar pattern with Faith by wanting, even expecting, her to do for herself what I was unwilling to do for myself. I hoped both of us could learn, in our own ways, how to answer the question: What is it to take responsibility for yourself? And I absolutely did not want her, twenty or thirty years from now, to be sitting in a therapist's office just like this one, unable to prioritize herself or her needs.

Kim watched me connect dots she'd been placing in front of me for months. "What would taking care of yourself look like?" she asked. "What would give you happi—"

"Happiness is overrated," I interrupted, pounding the couch cushion. "We've been sold a bill of goods about being happy all the time. Happiness is as fleeting as every other emotion. It makes more sense to seek." I paused, watching the candle flame dance. "Well, to seek contentment, peace."

Yes, Mary Pipher. Peace was what I was seeking too, and in this moment I was grasping for a way to understand connection to something deeper, more durable, to a way of being that went beyond the capriciousness of emotion and thought. I didn't know what that something was, but I sensed it existed. Or I hoped it existed.

"Okay," Kim said. "Then what would contentment look like, and how would that change your family dynamic?" Here we were, again, back to one person's effect on the whole.

Kim would probably have been satisfied with just about any answer. Learn to sail. Join a bowling league. But simple was not how I rolled.

"I guess that's what I have to figure out."

SPAGHETTI

Theo and I settled into The AG Center routine. Since our anniversary getaway, we'd been trying to be more tender with one another, patient. Every Wednesday, we drove downtown for family therapy and parent education classes. Every Saturday, for family group sessions and visiting time. The team was witnessing Faith's up and downs, working with her on understanding triggers and building coping skills, and she hit the one-month milestone living there. My fears about being abandoned again by people tasked with helping us were diminishing. Over the weeks, in addition to the wheel assignment, we discussed healthy boundaries, family structure, positive reinforcement, communication skills, and the nonlinear nature of recovery.

One evening, after parent education class, Theo pulled the car away from the curb. "They're giving us *a lot* of information," he said.

"It's like throwing spaghetti at the wall," I said.

"What do you mean?"

"They're hoping some of it will stick."

He had a point. But the volume of information was less stunning to me than the different ways Theo and I answered some of the questions. During the positive reinforcement workshop, for example, we were asked to write a list of Faith's top five negative behaviors. My top item: cutting. Theo's top item: profanity.

Seriously? After seventeen years of marriage, I wondered how he could still so consistently dismay and confuse me.

In family sessions, with Faith's newest therapist, Dr. June, Faith would sit on the couch between Theo and me, picking her cuticles. She was opening up more about the impact of my mom's death. "After Grandma, I'm scared about my mom or dad dying. What would happen to the other one? To me? What would we do? How would we survive?"

Rather than a cause of her illness, Theo and I were learning to understand Mom's death as a trigger. We would never fully understand how the two linked together. And in the long run, what to do to help Faith was far more important than dissecting the cause-effect link, the why.

She talked about other people. "No one is ever going to love me. I've gotta be perfect, keep everyone happy, but I screw everything up. I can't do anything right." I could certainly relate to feeling like that.

She talked about being bullied. "I never told anyone this, but in addition to being called names, the bullying got physical sometimes." Rage flooded my body as I thought back to the way Faith had said she hit her head to knock the bad thoughts out—that the truth was, very real and very cruel voices had seeded many of those thoughts. To my way of thinking, we'd given short shrift to bullying's impact on Faith's mental health.

And Faith talked about school. "I'm stressed and worried. I don't know how they'll treat me." She meant other students, and she obviously had ample reason to be afraid. When she was receptive, I'd wrap her in my arms, cuddle up close, or simply put my hand on her leg. When she wasn't, I honored the physical and emotional distance between us.

Dr. June emailed regular reports about Faith's progress, about the behavior they were witnessing and how they addressed her "dysregulation"—the clinical word for a biological process that gripped her mind, body, and soul. She shared about the work the staff was doing to help Faith process thoughts and feelings, calm down, and regulate. One day, in family session, Dr. June asked Faith to imagine life like a big bucket with a small hole in the bottom. "Put big chunks, like rocks, of love inside it," she said. "Because people do love you, Faith." At this, Faith nodded. "Your parents love you, the rest of your family, and friends. Try to imagine the hurt and fear like sand. Let it sift around the rocks and out the hole. Focus your concentration on what's left."

"I'll try," Faith said.

I'll try too, I thought.

FINDING THE SLACK

On the day Theo and I returned home from our anniversary trip to Ojai, I'd transferred the whole person wheel charts from my purse to a cabinet in my desk right next to where I sat to write, research, and make calls. Often, I peeked into the cabinet—white space glaring in the dimness representing my core belief that nothing I did was good enough. Ergo, I wasn't good enough.

I would close the cabinet door, cogitate, and wonder what to do. There was much to consider. Six different needs. Body. Brain. Spirit. Peace. Contentment. Where to begin? Friend? Gym? Guru? Could I trust myself not to screw up again? *It's too much*. Then I'd procrastinate by doing something else.

At my desk now, this was another one of those days. I peeked. Yep. My wheel, a.k.a. me, still needed an infusion of light and air, more balance.

I reflected on Mary Pipher's pronouncement that self-improvement projects are aggression. I'd been flagellating myself in the name of improvement for as long as I could remember, worse since Faith got sick. The negativity had done me exactly zero good. Had, it seemed in retrospect, driven me deeper inside myself behind even more layers of avoidance, isolation, and denial. On occasion, Kim and I discussed the purpose these reactions served: protection. But now, protection seemed to be another word for alone.

I thought about the untrue things Faith said about herself, the similarity of our charts, and Kim's gentle confrontation about the overblown meaning I'd made of one piece of paper. Ergo, again, perhaps the cruel words I said to myself were as untrue as the ones Faith said to herself. I was bone-weary of being so mean to myself. There had to be a better way.

What would it take for me to be kinder to myself? *More information*, I thought, per usual. In the future, I will learn that rumination and overthinking are common symptoms of a childhood like mine. But at this moment, I still assumed most folks' thoughts spun in a similar fashion.

I launched my computer browser, typed in "whole person wheel." Google's dropdown suggested the word "wellness," and a long list of websites populated my screen. I avoided government sponsored and wellness coach options, found a link whose language, about an individual's potentials, echoed the instructions we'd been given.

A center for successful aging, the banner read. Huh. I could see a graphic that listed the exact same six needs from our wheel: *spiritual, volitional, emotional, physical, social, intellectual*. The website explained that the woman who had created the model had done so for use in older-adult settings, like nursing homes and residential elder care facilities. I kept reading. "The principles of whole-person wellness help our clients maintain a lifestyle that is of the highest quality." No mention of mental illness, crappy mothering, or whipping asses into shape. In other words, the point of this therapeutic tool was to help seniors make the most of their twilight years. Or to help anyone increase their satisfaction and enthusiasm for life. I let out a long, loud breath.

These last many months, life/the universe/source/circumstance/whatever had presented me with what felt like one wake-up call after the next, leading me here. My cruelty was, in a word, unsustainable. Further: unnecessary. Even further:

the negativity had to be contaminating my relationships in ways I didn't understand.

Instantly, a weight lifted. My chest felt lighter. I realized the pain under my right shoulder blade had lessened. A new understanding, a different perspective entered my mind. I could view my white space as positive. In essence, flip the coin from tails to heads. My white space now overflowed with possibility. One hundred percent fulfillment had the potential to block growth. At one hundred percent fulfilled, what's left to explore? To learn? To try? Why even bother?

Maybe I was just wired differently than other folks. Faith too. My family of three was certainly resilient, still showing up, still figuring things out, and still supporting one another.

For the first time in a long while, I was excited about the future.

LAUREN PATRICE

I stared out the kitchen window. "We should box up the important stuff," I said. "Just in case."

Theo stood behind me, also staring out the window. "Don't overreact."

In the distance, flames were burning on Boney Peak's ridgeline; thick smoke billowed into the sky, obscuring sunshine with an ashy pall. Wind whipped our neighbor's palm fronds into a dizzying frenzy. Orange fire retardant streaked the hillside. It looked apocalyptic. Faith had been at The AG Center for five weeks, and for once I was relieved she wasn't home.

"I don't think it's overreacting when you can see flames out your window," I said.

California fires were nothing new, but this one's proximity to us was new, at least to me. It had erupted the prior day, and now about a mile north of us an entire housing community was being evacuated. Overnight and still, helicopters thundered to the burning areas that stretched from Camarillo to Newbury Park to the Pacific Coast Highway.

Theo grabbed the binoculars, headed for the front door. "I've lived here since the seventies, never had to evacuate."

"I hope we don't break that trend," I said.

He walked to the foot of the driveway, while I thought about the possibility of our home burning down. There was nothing to do but wait and see which way the wind would blow, literally.

I walked down the hall trying to prioritize a list of items should the need for a fast getaway arise. You think it'll be easy to decide, until you actually have to.

In the middle of our bedroom, I took in a 360-degree view. My wedding ring, in my jewelry box. Mom's treasures, in the bottom dresser drawer. Decades' worth of my photo albums lined the shelves. Important documents. Outside, fire burned, brittle wind gusted, another helicopter barreled by.

I noticed the edge of a plastic storage container under the bed. When Bob had arrived, in addition to having Mom's ashes and some family heirlooms, he'd brought two photo albums and a few other small odds and ends. In the rush of preparations, I'd stored everything in the box, shoved the box under the bed.

I sat on the floor, popped off the lid. On top, one of Mom's old photo albums, bright red. Suddenly, I was a one-year-old again. I hadn't seen those pictures in decades. Maybe ever. Dad, more pepper than salt in his crew cut, holding me, kissing my cheek, the way he always did. Dad's mom, smiling next to a handmade "Happy 70th Birthday" card. She would die a few years later. Chubby-cheeked me inside Mom's cherry-red car, a Pontiac Catalina. Determined-looking me on my glider horse exactly as serious as Faith had been on the one Mom had gotten for her. Mom was right about that. Our house on the lake, we had never once, rightly or wrongly, feared would burn down. But the memories seared, beautiful and hot.

On the second page, a family gathering in our backyard, next to the date 8-70, written in Mom's hand. August 1970 would have been my second birthday party. My eyes glided down the page. Dad, in gray shorts and a green T-shirt, is sitting in a chair in front of a picnic table. Mom, in white shorts and a blue-and-white blouse, her long brown hair held back in a barrette, perches precariously on one of his legs, one arm thrown around his shoulders. They both wear glasses. Mom's mouth is open, as if calling out. Maybe to me. Or to the photographer, whoever it was. But what I could not stop staring at was my mother's giant, pregnant belly.

In the past, present, and future, this photograph and one more like it will be the only evidence I know of that Lauren existed. The day she was born and also died must have occurred in September.

I heard the front door open. "I think we're going to be fine," Theo called down the hallway. "If I get nervous, I'll call Larry." Our neighbor was a retired fire chief.

I stared at Mom's belly, trying to make sense of how I could know and not know at all that I was supposed to have had a baby sister. But my whole life had been like that. Knowing and not at all knowing, maintaining the status quo. What did I remember? Dad, when I was very young, saying Lauren's name, once, telling me not to bring her up. All those times we escaped the house, which was us escaping my mother. My childhood was him and me, when it should have been Mom and Dad—a united couple—and a child. But what else did I remember?

One more memory. Mom and me. I was much older, had to be around sixteen. We were standing next to the formal dining table. Summer break was over, school had started, and we'd already celebrated Dad's birthday, so it was past the second of September. I remembered the feeling of tension building. Not unusual for my childhood. But the day I was remembering was worse than usual. Mom had been snippy with Dad, snippy with me. What she'd said to piss me off to the point of confrontation I could not recall.

What I'd said was, "What the hell is your problem?"

Mom had dropped whatever was in her hand, a pack of cigarettes, probably. "What's my problem? Today is your sister's birthday."

"Whose?" I'd said, at the split second I remembered.

"Your sister," Mom had said slowly and with what I'd taken to be contempt. Fourteen years had passed between Lauren's death and this exchange.

I probably said, "Oh," but it was already too late. Whatever window Mom had opened slammed shut, and she'd headed for the stairs, leaving me standing there. Thoughts along the lines of, *What do you expect? We never talk about her! It's not my fault. How was I supposed to know the date of her birthday/deathday?* Feeling rejected, I'd probably walked around for a while in a daze, coming up with ways to appease the pain I'd caused. Or maybe I'd shrugged, instantly forgetting again as Dad had instructed me years prior to do.

I flipped to the next page in the album. Christmas. Dad. Me. Mom. No big belly. No baby. Only the pretense that life was fine, because on the surface it was fine.

Lauren had come up once, at some point during my early therapy with Dolly, around the time she'd suggested my parents' actual problems had had little to do with me. No medical cause for my stomach aches and vomiting was uncovered, I'd explained. Together, we'd figured that throwing up had been my response to stress in the house.

I sat on the floor, the album still in my lap. I'd always vaguely understood Lauren's death as the beginning of the eventual end of my parents' marriage, not that anyone said so. Beyond that I had thought nothing about potential connections between Lauren and me. If I'd had the conscious thought to wonder, at sixteen years old, if Mom had wished Lauren had lived instead of me, if that was why I felt like sloppy seconds, if there was even more, much more, to the story than that, I couldn't say.

I put the album back in the plastic box, replaced the lid, and shoved it under the bed.

Back in the kitchen, I watched the flames burn.

FORGIVENESS

Six weeks after Faith arrived at The AG Center, she was slated soon to return home. But first, we had one final assignment to complete in family group therapy. Joel explained that being able to offer and receive forgiveness is an important part of recovery and healing. Our instructions: fill in the blanks on the "Forgiveness Script" and read them to one another out loud.

When it was our turn, Theo, Faith, and I walked to the middle of the room. Faith sat across from us: hesitant eyes, tight mouth, jouncing legs—a slight improvement over jackhammering. Theo volunteered to go first, clearing his throat. "Regarding the situation when you hurt yourself, I have been holding on to feeling angry and hurt. I am choosing to now forgive you for this experience. I forgive you."

He nodded at Faith who blushed, her expression softening.

"My turn," I said, without hesitation. "Regarding the situation when you cut yourself and lied about it, I have been holding on to feelings of fear, anger, and pain." My voice quivered a little, but not too bad. "I am choosing to now forgive you for this experience. I forgive you." I smiled, hoping she felt my sincerity.

Faith raised her paper. "Regarding the situation when you made me feel bad about cutting, purging, or restricting, I have been holding on to feelings of guilt and pain. I am choosing to now forgive you. I forgive you." She lowered the paper enough to peer over the top at Theo and me.

"Thanks, babe," I said. My insides felt squishy. "I love you."

"I love you too, Mom." She looked at Theo. "I love you, Dad."

"I love you too, baby doll," he said.

"Any thoughts on that?" Joel asked.

"Yeah," I said, jumping in. "Of course, as a mom, I've forgiven Faith during every step of this process. Nothing about this is her fault, but I never thought about saying I forgive her out loud. Saying so never even crossed my mind. How would she know if I never told her? And vice versa. Doing this together helped me feel closer to her and also see my actions in a new way, from her point of view." I paused. "I mean, just because I feel my reactions were normal, I understand more clearly that they still had a negative impact on Faith."

Joel smiled. "Good job, Yokases."

I beamed, still a sucker for approval.

Joel handed each of us a small red glass bead—a token to remember the day by. I stuck mine in my pocket for safekeeping.

We moved aside so the next family could take the hot seats. As they read their statements, my thoughts wandered. The idea was stupidly simple: say out loud the words, "I forgive you." How had I never thought of that?

I had no trouble telling Faith I loved her, but conversations around the harder emotions? They were usually Theo and me talking, Faith listening, and us minimizing her feelings. Or full-on arguments. And I'd dismissed as unimportant conflicts over cell phones and Facebook accounts even though they were important to her. However inadvertently, it was clearer now that Theo and I had, in word and deed, and in lack of word and deed, been hurting each other and Faith.

I didn't expect us to never hurt or offend one another again. No. This assignment demonstrated the point that ruptures require the work of repair.

"I forgive you," said the mom in the middle of the room to her son.

Repair. Into my mind popped a habit of Mom's, signing off from phone calls with me by saying, "Love ya." Never using the full three words. I wondered if she'd noticed she did that, because I sure had. Whenever Mom said, "Love ya," I'd mimicked her with a singsongy response, "Love ya too." One memory. On a beach, waves rolling in, infant Faith asleep in the stroller, Mom and I staring out at the ocean, large conch shells rolling around at our feet. "I love you," Mom had finally said—post–all-you-could-drink champagne breakfast buffet.

After that, my sarcasm had morphed into melancholy, and whenever she'd say, "Love ya," I would simply say, "You too."

The boy, across from his mom, said, "I forgive you."

Why hadn't I asked my mother about saying, "I love you"? I could guess, after everything we'd now been through with Faith, after everything I'd read, and after everything I kept learning, that the answer was simple. And complex: I'd never learned how. My parents had never, to my knowledge, had these discussions with each other. Nor with me. No "I'm sorry." No "I forgive you." No "Please forgive me."

Had that been what Mom had wished for, lying in a hospital bed, unable to speak, with longing on her face? After so many years, had she finally wanted me to know, clearly, unequivocally, that she loved me? At least the full phrase was the last words she'd heard me say.

Faith sat beside me. I looked at her, yearning. I recognized the pattern: unspoken words between mother and daughter. I wanted to change that dynamic with Faith. Wanted her to know we could talk about anything. Everything. All the things I'd not thought to say. All the things she'd not thought to ask. There was time. I could improve my communication with Faith. Theo and other people too.

THE SNAG

Mere days before Faith was supposed to come home, we hit a snag. Dr. June reported that Faith's behavior had deteriorated. Via a combination of emails, phone calls, and an in-person meeting, Dr. June said Faith was scratching herself, swearing, and being verbally aggressive toward the staff—the pattern of self-sabotage had reemerged. "I asked her about it," Dr. June said, "and her response was basically, 'What do you expect, my grandmother died.'"

Dr. June said she was working to move Faith toward the resolution stage of grief, where she could acknowledge missing her grandmother and know that she'd be okay. I wondered what she meant exactly by "moving toward resolution," because her words suggested an agency over this process that no one had so far had.

Joel, the primary therapist, proposed we postpone graduation. I wanted to punch him. Then, I wanted to proceed on schedule. Theo was working a freelance gig, gone every day again from very early until very late, and said he'd go along with whatever was decided. I petitioned Dr. June and Joel, reminding them, in lengthy and detailed emails, that we were ready for every contingency. A thorough plan was in place, again. "All three of us have learned and grown," I said. And, I reminded them, once the testing phase of the IEP was completed, we'd have access to even more support through the school district.

At the last minute, we got the green light, with the caveat that the success of Faith's graduation from the program, huge as it was, would not guarantee abstinence at home from disordered eating or self-harm. In fact, Dr. June and Joel said we should count on seeing those behaviors emerge whenever Faith felt overwhelmed, chaotic, and out of control. They reminded me that recovery is nonlinear and that Faith's ability to stay home would depend on slips being "reasonable." Theo and I needed to remain calm, keep our expectations in check.

BATTLE ARMOR, KIT ADDITIONS

Notes on goodbye, thank you
Nonviolent Communication, by Marshall Rosenberg

HOME, AGAIN

Seven weeks after Faith arrived at AG, we drove home together on a Saturday. She walked straight to her room, perked up instantly. "Oh, my god!" she said, taking in Theo's completed handiwork: eggplant paint, zebra-striped wallpaper.

"I'm glad you like it," Theo said. He'd worked hard to accomplish her specific requests.

She plopped into the zebra-striped bean bag chair, squirmed around, then rolled off onto the soft, clean zebra-striped throw rug. "I want to order some posters and stuff to put up."

"Your room, your walls," I said.

"I've got lots of duct tape," Theo said.

Off to a good start! I carried Faith's suitcase to the garage. She'd mentioned seeing cockroaches at the center—a part of treatment I definitely planned to leave behind.

Three days later, Faith approached me about ridding her room of "little kid stuff."

"Great idea," I said. "Let's do it."

I grabbed several clean garbage bags, thought immediately of that awful Dr. Amanda. A burst of anger flooded my chest. I felt like calling her, reaming her out, elucidating details of people who actually cared and tried to be helpful. Instead, in Faith's room, we purged. The good kind.

We started with the closet, rifling through clothes, folding donations, filling one bag and then another. We emptied drawers. Bubble-wrapped knickknacks. Stacked old games and toys. Collected outgrown sports gear. I scooped an armload of stuffed animals out of the hot-pink plastic baby doll crib.

"We'll have to sort through these," I said, dumping bunnies, monkeys, seals, lions, and bears onto the floor. Many were gifts from special people, including my mother, with which we would not part.

"Okay," Faith said, busy with a rack of bins across the room.

I scooped, dug, and dumped out the remaining animals. At the bottom of the crib, under the last furry friend, lay a serrated steak knife.

I bent in half, taking in the inert silver blade, black resin handle, faint reddish-brown stains. I stared harder at the stains: old. The knife looked strange against the vibrant, babyish fabric. Ghoulish. I vaguely remembered noticing a while ago that a steak knife was missing from the kitchen drawer, had promptly forgotten about it. Later, we'd locked them up. This knife must have been in the crib for months.

I didn't want to shame or upset Faith. I thought about trying to hide the knife under my shirt, in my pants. Options that seemed disingenuous. There was nothing else to do. Calmly, I picked the knife up, turned. Faith noticed me, my hand. We said nothing: no freaking out, no accusations, no denials.

Alone at the kitchen sink, I inspected the blade's dips and points, the fine edge. With everything that had happened over the last few months, Faith had probably forgotten about it too. I dropped the knife into the dishwasher, hoping no more surprise discoveries lay in store.

GUARDRAILS

The new plan we'd crafted for Faith's return home was a lot like the old plan.

Every week, she would meet twice with Mona, her first therapist, for talk therapy and twice with a tutor for math and English schoolwork. Once a week, she'd meet with the nutritionist for meal planning and a therapist trainee would come to the house to help her work on emotions in her home environment. Once a month, she'd see a psychiatrist for a medication review. A few light chores, like doing her laundry and vacuuming. Faith would earn privileges, like time to hang out with friends or be on her cell phone, dependent on a collaborative attitude and abstinence from harmful behavior. So that she'd always know what was happening and when, we devised a color-coded schedule to account for meal times, appointments, errands, exercise time, fun with friends, and whatever else would be necessary.

There was also a separate, written safety plan that outlined Theo's and my actions and responsibilities in the event of a serious self-harm incident, and Faith had signed off on it. Soon, her beloved summer drama program would start. Performing brought out the best in Faith, and she needed the confidence boost, the community, to be involved in something bigger than herself—purpose and meaning. The program director, who'd known Faith since second grade, adored her, and would, I knew, keep a nuanced eye on one of her favorite performers.

The guardrails were in place, and we reached five days and then beyond with no call to 911.

Faith was relieved to be home, and still had trouble settling in. Not surprising. Altogether, she'd been gone for the better part of three months; it was now May. During the week, her friends were still in school, but on the weekends, Faith was now joining in for trips to the beach, a movie, or the local street fair. I heard laughter, saw flashes of Faith's former smile. I made use of her short stints away from home to again check drawers, cabinets, and nooks and crannies. She wanted us to trust her, and I wanted to trust her, but it was too soon. Sentiments Faith would sometimes express sounded like: "I feel trapped here. My friends and the cat are the most important things to me. I miss cutting." Instead of rolling my eyes or sighing, I said, "I understand." Because I did. Finally.

A coping skill is a coping skill, and how much better were mine? Who was I to judge?

During the day, Faith refused my hugs. No more cuddles watching TV. Age appropriate, of course. But I missed having her in my arms. At night, she had nightmares, would scream, causing Theo and me to jolt awake with fear and dread. Our hearts pounding, one of us would run to her room, stroke her hair, murmur calm words, straighten her comforter, and kiss her forehead. She'd roll over and go back to sleep, but we'd lie down and spin out, waiting for our pulse rates to return to normal.

Theo and I, in a therapy session, not with Faith present, expressed feeling a constant mid- to high-grade apprehension that something would trigger another severe downward spiral—reasonable reactions for which we alone were responsible. Whichever therapist we were with used an earthquake analogy.

"You're waiting to see how long, how serious, and what the aftershocks will be like." Having been in a couple of real earthquakes, I concurred.

I reminded myself to take each day as it came, had not forgotten about my pie chart, or the insights I'd gleaned, or about wanting to talk more with Faith. But the fact of the matter was, we weren't ready yet for those types of conversations. Healing requires steps forward and backward, and we were busy enough managing daily life.

When dysregulation happened, because of course it did, Faith would cry. In her bedroom or the living room, she might fall to the floor, curl into a ball, and wail—painful thoughts, feelings, and emotions pouring out of her. If Theo was home, I ordered him to the garage and he'd usually comply. Progress. Instead of reacting in fear, despair, and confusion, now (at least on the outside) I could respond differently.

Calmness—concerted and focused—had required discussion with the therapists, input from Faith, trial and error, and lots of practice, for which life afforded me opportunity. Over time, I improved. I learned to sit on the floor, breathe, remain quiet and very still, preventing my own body and my own emotions from being hijacked. *We are two different people*, I reminded myself. Disentangle. *Faith's her own person. I'm separate from her. Those are her feelings, not mine. I'm okay even if she isn't right now. I can be here for her.* I thought these words like a mantra, over and over again.

I could witness Faith's pain, without trying, at least most of the time, to intervene or to fix, without floating away on waves of my own anxiety, without being swept up in currents of fear. It made complete sense to feel terrible when she felt terrible. Pithy quip: A parent is only as happy as their least happy child. But that dynamic, exactly, was what required my attention.

Sweaty and spent, Faith would calm down, because she would

always eventually calm down. Occasionally, when she wanted to, we'd talk about what had upset her—usually something to do with school. But often she was too exhausted for words, and I'd encourage her to recuperate with rest, sleep, music, art, or by watching a lighthearted TV show.

When the worst of her distress passed, if she was receptive, like at the treatment center, I might put my hand on her leg or rub her back. If she wasn't, I sat. Waited. I was learning how to be a safe space, gratified that my hard work was starting to pay off.

The urge to fix was powerful and still swelled inside me, but again, with practice and attention I learned how to recognize the feeling, breathe through it, and remain present and alert. Wanting to fix implies brokenness, incapacity. My daughter wasn't broken. She was not "too much." And she needed to know her mother had her back.

AS PREDICTED

Soiled tissues, dirty Band-Aids
Less often, less seriously
Yeah, sometimes we were calmer.
And still upset, angry, disappointed, frustrated, and confused.
And still making progress.

THE SECRET SAUCE

Halfway through the summer after Faith came home, in July, I sat with Kim for my weekly session. She knew disruptive and self-harming behavior had returned, kept reminding me it was a normal part of the recovery process. This was still early in my work learning to be a calmer, truer version of myself, and some days I was better at accepting normal recovery than others. This day, as I recounted a recent excursion with Faith and a couple of her friends, I was feeling sorry for myself.

"How'd it go at the beach?" Kim asked.

"Pretty good, I guess, but I think Faith's oversharing about her experiences in treatment. I suggested to her later that she might want to keep some things private."

"Is that for her sake or yours?"

"Both, I guess."

"A natural consequence might work better."

I tucked that thought away for later. "Drama's going well," I said. "Faith got the lead, again, but the one-year anniversary of my mom's death is coming up."

"Oh, wow. Already? How are you feeling about that?"

"I don't know. Most days are a blur, but when I have time to think about it, I'm just sad. And scared. With all I've learned, I'm still worried about Faith and me, because, honestly, I'm tired."

Kim frowned. "The attitude, the . . ."—I hesitated—"rest. I bet she feels the same way."

"What are you doing for yourself?" Kim asked.

"What *can* I do?" I said, shrugging. "I have to be available at a moment's notice in case anyone needs something. I'm trying to take responsibility for my stuff, stay positive. I've done it all and here we are. There's nothing left to try."

"You could try having some compassion for your daughter," Kim said.

"What?" I asked, confused, my body suddenly stiff. "If I'm not the compassionate one in this equation, who is?"

ONE-YEAR ANNIVERSARY

I kicked off my flip-flops, sank my feet into the soft, warm sand. Faith stood beside me. Waves rolled onto the shoreline. July 20, 2013. The one-year anniversary of Mom's death, a couple of weeks after that session with Kim. Along with Mom's partner, Bob, who'd flown in from New Jersey, Theo, Faith, and I were at the beach to pay tribute to Mom. It was Saturday. Families, couples, people walking their dogs, blankets, coolers, and umbrellas dotted the landscape.

Theo and Bob set up beach chairs. Faith and I turned around, our shadows shortish and roundish in the midday sun. Faith unfurled her towel, placed it right next to mine. She peeled off her top and shorts down to her bathing suit. Her weight still looked to be more or less holding steady. A breeze rustled her hair. Nearby, a family building a castle reminded me of the days when Theo would bring a shovel and dig a giant hole. Kids, playing tag with the waves, screeched with glee, just like Faith had done at that age.

As she folded her clothes, I caught a glimpse of a scar, felt awash in gratitude for her health, her life, for what we'd survived, our resilience and ability to be together on this day.

I pointed to our beach bag. "Sunscreen," I said to Faith.

"Don't need it," she said.

I was already slathered, of course, a giant floppy hat shading my face and shoulders. "I know, but use it anyway, please. You know how much you hate a sunburn."

She acquiesced, and the hiss of the aerosol can sent the chemical smell drifting my way. "I miss Grandma," she said.

"I do too, love," I said. And it was true. Most of all, I missed what might have been. "She'd be so proud of you, though. She *is* so proud of you."

Sunlight danced on the water's crests and troughs; colors shifted from white to turquoise to deep blue. As soon as the beach had hit our sight line, Faith had relaxed—kindred souls, she and Grandma, in their love for the ocean.

Bob stood. "I'll be back." He headed toward the water's edge, his own footprints following along behind him.

I guessed he wanted to reminisce in private. We hadn't seen him since the previous year, when he'd driven out with Mom's ashes. It must have been as strange for him as it was for us, being together without her.

Faith lay beside me, soaking up the sun. Theo was reading. I ran my fingers through the fine, soft sand. I scooped some up and let it sift from my hand. I'd been journal writing, reading, thinking, and talking more to Kim about compassion, and I'd realized that she was right. Again. I'd been mistaking an unhealthy tendency of self-sacrifice and pragmatic parts of the journey, like scheduling appointments and doing research, as compassionate acts that would, at least theoretically, lessen Faith's suffering—a tiny sliver of a much larger truth.

Compassion in action is actually a set of skills. Skills I'd never learned, requiring an ability to connect, in the fullest sense, with empathy, kindness, and understanding to our shared human experience. Similar to how I'd never learned how to repair communication, talk about difficult feelings, or set healthy boundaries. But therein lay the rub: in order to connect to anyone else in compassion, I first had to connect that way with myself.

Faith sat up. Sweat beaded on her forehead, trickled down the sides of her face. "I'm going in," she said.

In another lifetime, a mermaid. "Enjoy," I said.

She hopped across the hot sand. Theo closed his book. "You okay?"

"Yeah, just sad," I said.

"All you have to do is think of your mother, and she'll be here."

"I know. Thank you."

Waves bandied Faith about like Gumby in the wind. She dove headlong into an oncoming swell, popped up on the other side, and flipped over to float on her back. I spotted Bob's outline, the size of a Lego, down the beach. In light of the last year, everything I used to admire about myself—sarcasm, perfectionism, overachieving—now seemed so . . . harsh. Critical. Judgmental. Fake.

Bob returned with Faith hot on his heels. She smelled of salt and seaweed. "Here," she said, dropping a few shells on my towel.

"Pretty, babe," I said.

"Should we do the flowers?" Bob asked.

I'd brought a small bouquet of carnations and unwrapped them now, releasing their sweet scent. I handed a single flower to Theo, Faith, and Bob, and kept one for myself.

At the water's edge, we spoke about my mom, Lauraine: mom, grandmother, partner, friend, survivor, *vilomah*—parent whose child died. Only now, for the first time, woman to woman, did I wish I could tell Lauraine how sorry I was about the death of her daughter, Lauren. That whatever her deficiencies in mothering me, around which there would be much more to uncover and to heal, I saw she had loved, lost, and grieved. I sensed a softening toward Mom, as a person who had not had the capacity, for whatever reason, to recognize or acknowledge the repercussions of our bloodlines.

Bob spoke first, finishing with, “You never know what you’ve got until it’s gone.”

Theo probably said, “May her memory be eternal.”

Faith said, “I miss you, Grandma.”

And me. I said, “I miss you, Mom. I love you.”

Foamy residue swirled around our feet. “Ready, guys?” I said. “One, two, three!”

We tossed our flowers into the sea.

FIRST DAY OF HIGH SCHOOL

I was staring out the kitchen window, admiring the inky outline of Boney Peak, stalwart regardless of whatever Mother Nature hurled its way. Faith's alarm echoed down the hallway. Twelve weeks after she'd returned home from residential treatment, today was the day. An official high school kid.

Faith joined me in the kitchen, sleep-mussed hair hanging in her eyes.

"Morning, love, how ya doing?" I asked.

"Okay," she yawned. Then she grabbed a box of cereal.

"Big day today," I said.

"Yep." She opened the fridge, dumped milk into the bowl.

"Don't forget your pills."

"I won't."

I was nervous, figured she was too. She hadn't been in a classroom for nine months. Grades wouldn't be a problem, but the rest?

Faith had mentioned maybe wanting to join the water polo team. My thoughts drifted, imagining so many teenage girls, together, in a locker room. *Stop. Stay here. Don't get ahead of yourself.* I'd been paying more attention to my habit of ruminating about the past or the future, missing out on what was happening right in front of me.

"What do you want for lunch today?"

"Just a sandwich." She gulped the last bit of milk from her bowl. "I've got to get ready."

I carried the paper bag down the hallway. Faith was in her bathroom, crafting the perfect cat-eye makeup look with liquid eyeliner. I lingered in the doorway watching her layer mascara on her lashes.

"What?" she said.

"Nothing." *Everything.*

I held up the bag. "I'll put this by your backpack."

When it was time, I zipped my sweatshirt over my pajama top. Faith came out of her room— cat-eyes, cute new outfit, and Claddagh ring from our trip when she was ten years old to Ireland. She slung her backpack over her shoulder. "Let's go," she said.

Faith was quiet as we drove past Albertson's. By Trader Joe's, I said, "I'll be home all day if you need anything."

"Okay, thanks. I think I'll be fine."

I pulled into the turn lane. In front of us, students streamed onto campus.

"You got this," I said. "You'll do great." I inched the car along the queue. Finally, we got to the curb. "Give me a hug. I'll be right here waiting for you after school."

"I love you, Mom."

"I love you too, babe."

She hopped out—fake diamonds in her triple-pierced ears glittered in the morning sunshine—and grabbed her backpack. I waved, watching her walk away. A team of people, including her dad and me, would facilitate whatever we could to help Faith. The rest was in her hands. I sat there until she disappeared from view.

At home, I raced to my journal. I never wanted to forget how overwhelmingly filled with gratitude I was, just to drop Faith off at school.

Each stroke of my pen awakened more joy, more ecstasy over

this "boring," "ordinary," "normal" moment. My daughter was a freshman in high school, like the rest of her friends. My hand was flying across the paper. Finn, lying in a patch of sunlight, stretched. Amazing! The pen, rubbing against my fingers, chafed. Glorious!

My phone rang. It was Isabelle's mom, Grace. I swiped to answer the call. She invited me to grab breakfast the next morning.

"Yes," I said. "Sounds great."

REPAIR

The details don't matter.

"I'm sorry," I said to my daughter, because I was sorry. I'd said or done something that required repair, an apology.

"I'm sorry too," she said.

"Thanks, but you've done nothing wrong," I said, because she hadn't. "You have nothing to apologize for."

Another day.

"I'm sorry," Faith said, because she was sorry. She'd said or done something that required repair, an apology.

"I accept," I said. "Thank you. I love you."

"I love you too," she said.

WITNESS

Faith, in her room, was doing homework and listening to that damn heavy metal music. Theo had fallen asleep on the couch. I was reading in bed. Three months into the school year, appearances indicated a return to ordinary in the Yokas household.

But all day, my gut had been on alert. Faith was upset about something. A cute boy, a sophomore named Benji, had asked Faith out and she'd said yes. A few weeks into their romance, she remained convinced he would soon break it off. I'd followed the therapists' instructions. "I love you," I'd said. "I'm here if you want to talk." She'd nodded. Nothing had come of it. Now, I was drowsy, about to ask her to turn down the music.

Her phone: *Bzz bzz, bzz-bzz.*

I sat up and looked across the hall. She was lying on the floor, propped up on her elbows. She returned the text.

I was about to call out when Faith put her phone down, picked up something else. She ran her right hand to the crook of her left arm, flicked. Then she dabbed at the spot with a crumpled black T-shirt.

I realized with a jolt she had just cut herself.

My heart pounded. My temples throbbed. *Are you kidding me?*

She hadn't noticed me, and I froze, watching, as she did it again.

I leaned back against my headboard. Limbs leaden. Until now, I'd never witnessed the behavior firsthand. Commentary ran through my mind: *Don't get into a power struggle. If she wants to cut, she will. Witness her pain. Remain calm. Be compassionate.*

For a split second, I thought about rolling over, turning out the light, and pretending not to know. Unacceptable. This situation required appropriate action. Compassion calls for courage. I was the adult, Faith my child. More than that: she was a fellow human being who hurt. I rubbed my palms against the comforter, took a deep breath, and tossed off the covers.

I sat on the edge of the bed. *My love is unconditional. You can do this. Be firm and kind.* Compassion calls for empathy.

I walked across the hall.

"Faith," I said—speaking louder than the screeching music, but not screaming.

She ignored me.

I kneeled down. Used my calm voice. "You're hurting yourself, please stop."

"No," she said, refusing to meet my eyes. "Leave me alone and get out."

I scanned the floor but saw no blade. Her fingers flew over the keypad of her cell phone.

"Please stop. Now."

"GET OUT!"

Anger flared. Before I could stop the thought: G*o ahead and cut your arm off.*

Seconds ticked by. My body vibrated, able to understand what my brain couldn't acknowledge. No amount of magical thinking would change the reality that Faith was in charge of her recovery. I stood up, walked away.

Back in bed: *What have I done?* I'd warned myself to avoid expectations, to take one day at a time. Faith had been doing well, and expectations had crept back in. And yes, goddamn it. I wanted her to stop cutting. Was that so wrong?

I breathed in through my nose and out through my mouth. Once, twice, three times. My heart rate slowed. I rubbed my palms, again, on the comforter. Looked straight ahead at the fanciful painting on the wall—a giant cat, Fuzzy, with a big fish hanging from its mouth. I stayed still, noticing blue water, pink scales, and green fur. Quiet. Compassion calls for mindfulness.

More purposeful thinking came back online. My reaction may have lacked finesse, but it was an improvement from the past. "Progress, not perfection," Theo might say, quoting a twelve-step motto, and he'd be right.

No matter what happened next, I'd be there for Faith. Compassion calls for forgiveness. I waited for the guilt to come, the inadequacy. Instead, *You're doing the best you can and it's enough*.

Then I felt peace.

"Mom," Faith called out, startling me. "I need you."

Fifteen minutes had passed. I rushed to her room.

"I can't stop the bleeding." She was clamping the black T-shirt down against her arm. Panic clouded her eyes.

She balled up like a turtle, started rocking back and forth.

I turned off the radio. Slid her phone out of my way, revealing a razor blade. Faith grabbed it, keening.

"I won't take it," I said, calmly. "I promise."

Theo appeared in the doorway. "What's going on?"

"She's upset," I said.

I punched up the contact list on Faith's phone, tapped the entry for her newest therapist.

"Terri." I handed Faith the phone.

One hour later, our crisis was over. Faith had spoken to Terri and had gone to sleep. Theo had returned to the living room. I'd climbed back into bed. Monday morning, I would follow protocol and alert the rest of the team, including the school psychologist and IEP personnel, so they could work through with Faith what had happened and why. By now, she would have re-hidden the razor blade somewhere in her room. I wasn't going to pillage or plunder to find it.

I inhaled. I exhaled. I noticed the coolness of my fingers, the air flowing in and out of my nose, and the softness inhabiting my body.

THE BIG FLUSH

It was Valentine's Day. Faith's first one with a real, live valentine. She was fifteen years old now and still together with Benji. We'd spent weeks planning a special day. We'd cleaned, cooked, and baked. We'd eaten. They were adorable, canoodling. I'd offered to do the dishes. Theo was still at work. Now it was 10 p.m.

Faith called from down the hallway. "Mom, can you come here?"

"Be right there."

Faith and Benji were standing in the doorway of her bathroom. "What's up, babe?" I asked, suddenly worried.

"I wanted you to see this." She was gazing into Benji's eyes.

"See what?"

Faith tilted her head toward the toilet. I squished between the two of them. A razor blade sat on the bottom of the bowl. I didn't want to move. I didn't want to breathe.

Faith flushed the toilet. Together, we watched the blade disappear.

I stepped back, stunned. "Thank you for sharing that with me," I said.

Faith and Benji hugged. I rubbed her back, felt, suddenly, like an intruder and headed for the living room. But at the end of the hallway, I turned around. Encircled in his arms, Faith gently kissed Benji on the lips. I figured she'd flushed the blade for him, and that was okay by me.

If our lives had been different leading up to that sweet kiss, I probably wouldn't have seen it or the hug. Or, knowing myself, I would have taken those simple acts for granted. But everything we'd done had led to this moment. I sent thanks to the universe, and I walked away to leave them to it.

GRATITUDE

Compassion calls for gratitude.

Before our healing journey, I paid no attention to gratitude—in fact, I found the idea of an "attitude of gratitude" schmaltzy. Then Faith received a diagnosis. I read somewhere that we're hungry for joy because we're starving from a lack of gratitude. When I'd read those words, I thought about the taking for granted I'd done of ordinary beauty. On the first day of Faith's freshman year of high school, as my hand raced across my journal, a veil had dropped from my eyes. Hitting my personal rock bottom and working my way back enabled me to notice what had always been right in front of me: abundance.

I wanted to bolster my new habit of noticing, to keep noticing and harness more joy. To that end, I created a simple daily practice. A small ritual. At bedtime, I reviewed the day and in a cheap notepad from a dollar store wrote down three things I was grateful for. I didn't mull or over-analyze, just jotted down whatever came to mind. I encouraged myself to think small, because small details—or what might seem small, anyway—were the easiest to overlook.

In bed, leaning against my pillow, I'd close my eyes. There was Faith, in her polo team bathing suit, jumping in the pool, water cascading off her face. There was Theo, going above and beyond to keep our lives running smoothly. There was my cat, who I loved like a human. I'd open my eyes, begin. Water polo goal! Theo, at the sewing machine! Finn's fur! I might write a word or two about why I was grateful for those things. Tenacity, new curtains, softness! The process usually took less than five minutes.

Soon, I noticed my perceptions shifting, again. A pink flower was actually fuchsia, vanilla coffee creamer tasted vanilla-ier, and Finn's black fur was actually black, blue, and silver. Outside, birdsong in trills and swirls. And man oh man, the smell when they cut the grass at a nearby park. The attention to detail made everything old brand-new. Noticing the aliveness around me, especially in nature, I felt connected to everything and everyone.

Transformation was working its way out of me from the inside.

CONSCIOUS CHOICE

Weight Watchers, again.

Wednesday, not Saturday.

Some lady, not Dolly.

Change of pace, I'd thought, in an effort to finally conquer the divide between me and my body.

Kicking off my sneakers, again.

Weighing in, again, heavier even than last time.

Taking a seat, I recognized the negativity enveloping me. The cover of the Weight Watchers weekly pamphlet in my hand read: *Get happy!* Exactly.

Scales. Food. Insults. They were the how, not the why. The self-improvement project of weight loss as a path to lasting happiness, of any external enterprise as a path to lasting happiness, was a dangerous lie, and always had been. An observable shift was happening inside me, making space. But not for looking on the bright side or finding something to be happy about.

A conscious choice: *I AM NOT DOING THIS TO MYSELF AGAIN. I am enough. And I acknowledge you, negative messaging. I feel you, inner sadness. I see you, low self-esteem. I honor your attempts to protect me. Thank you.*

I could be content with my body *and* I could accept that too much weight was suboptimal. I wasn't in denial. I was changing.

I had no idea where the conscious choice to start loving myself unconditionally would lead, and that was okay. I didn't need to know.

Hello, breaking a pattern. Goodbye, Weight Watchers.

A WHOLE PERSON WHEEL, REDESIGNED

The problem with the pie chart was its shape.

Rather than a hole or a circle at the center, the slices converged in the middle to a point. In other words, the wheel had no hub, no opening, nothing at its core that stabilized the larger whole.

There are no wrong choices in a healing journey, just each next one. Or a choice at any given moment not to choose, to wait, be still, and open to intuition.

Awareness—dedication to making conscious choices, waking up—at the center of wholeness moves me away from reactivity and toward response. This is how I take responsibility for myself.

THE SCAR

I was six years old, in the kitchen with Dad. He was on the phone. Mom was out of town, and it was time for *The Six Million Dollar Man* to start. Dad just kept talking and talking, so I ran. I didn't want to miss it. I ran as fast as my bionic legs could carry me. Faster than a car.

I streaked out of the kitchen, my nightgown fluttering behind me, past the dining table, onto the shaggy carpet, past Bumpy. But I tripped. And my head bashed right into the pointed knob for changing the channel. Back then, televisions had sharp, pointy knobs.

I screamed. Could see only red. Blood poured out of my head covering both my eyes, falling onto my legs. I screamed and screamed.

Dad scooped me up. Then I was in the emergency room. I was lying down, and they covered my face with a cloth. I tried not to cry, but the thing I loved most had hurt me.

As a doctor pierced a needle through my skin and sewed my forehead back together, Dad held my hand. He told me what a brave big girl I was. It didn't really hurt anymore, they'd given me medicine, but I could feel the tugging and pulling, my forehead moving, skin stretching. I thought I might throw up. Turned out, the horizontal cut was an inch long, and at the exact spot where skin met hair.

At home, for days, I sat on Dad's lap. When my stitches hurt, he got a damp cloth. He told me not to touch them so they wouldn't get dirty. I did my part. He worked hard to make me comfortable. I worked hard too. I was sitting on his lap when Mom walked through the front door. I remember the *Oh, my god, what happened now?* look on her face, but not what Dad said.

People used to ask me, when my hair was pulled back, what had happened to my head. For many years the scar was obvious, and I'd tell the story, recalling the surprise, the pain, the confusion, the teamwork. Laughing a little: my head + a television = the irony. Then, years later, the scar was suddenly all but gone.

Now, I am the only person who can find the barely there line. Most of the time, I forget I even have a scar. When I look for it, I see a reminder that certain of life's circumstances are indisputable, and yet. The greatest connections are forged by our choices. In that barely there line, I see my superpower. Steve Austin may have had a bionic eye, but I have aligned past and present.

Carrying forward remnants of my history, I continue to shift.

EPILOGUE

I stood over my art journal, in the office at home, dripping drops of watermelon-red alcohol ink onto a layer of dry, white gesso. A beam of sunshine shone through the skylight, creating a bright white patch on the hardwood floor. Inside the warm glow, Finn lay sleeping.

It was summer. Faith had completed her freshman year of high school with the same boyfriend, a water polo coaches' award, and on the honor roll. Theo and I were proud of her dedication. Now, she was at drama camp, rehearsing her part as Scarecrow in *The Wizard of Oz*. The gift of song was back in the house.

Next to the red ink, I added some drops of sailboat blue and citrus green. An acrid odor wafted into my nostrils. I'd seen this particular technique on YouTube, searching mixed media videos. Using a straw, I blew the wet ink around the page. Watermelons, sailboats, and citruses spidered across the page, droplets morphing into what looked like colorful zaps of lightning.

The process was flawed, I knew. Alcohol ink works best on a specific type of slick polypropylene paper called Yupo. I had none, but no one would know if I made a mistake. Or if what I made was ugly. This play was only for me. Fun on my own terms.

My return to a creative practice had started about seven months prior to this with a book, of course. And permission. I'd read Brené Brown's *The Gifts of Imperfection*. In the section about creativity, Brown wrote that contrary to what we may have been taught, human beings are inherently creative, need, in fact, to express ourselves through art. As I'd read those words, I'd remembered joyful moments from my childhood and from Faith's. Time spent singing, dancing, and writing, or hunched over drawing pads and coloring books with pencils, crayons, and markers. Deep in my gut, a tickle-like sensation had formed, spreading up and out to my fingers. They'd itched with longing for color, shape, texture, imagery.

Reclaim what you loved, the feeling had seemed to indicate. Faith had been holding her own in school, the guardrails sturdy and strong, withstanding bumps and dings. In between appointments, IEP meetings, and water polo matches, I'd finally felt ready for a deeper dive into self-care, for a way of tending to myself that went beyond adequate hydration, Swedish massage, and even therapy appointments. Following Brené's advice to give myself permission to do what I needed to do, I'd enrolled in an online class, armed with Post-it Notes, old markers, broken crayons, some Sharpies, and her words, "I'm imperfect and I'm enough."

I'd had no idea what I was doing, but that hadn't mattered. Onto the white paper, I'd layered images cut from magazines, words printed from my computer, and stickers (cats and butterflies) from the bottom of Faith's toy chest. I'd drawn childlike flowers with green spiky leaves, had raided Theo's work box for patterned duct tape (peace signs!), and had colored crayon rainbows. Soon, to satisfy a growing craving, I'd needed more supplies.

So I'd ordered Mod Podge, glue sticks, acrylic paint, brushes, watercolors, and glitter. I'd trolled the aisles at JoAnn Fabrics and Michael's, finding paper pads, washi tape, and an adult mandala coloring book. I'd asked Theo, who was ogling my amassing stash, to fetch a table from storage. "I need to add on to the house!" he'd said with a smile, supportive.

EPILOGUE

Day after day, for five minutes or for an hour, I'd kept watching videos, making pages. Typing into the computer quotes about boundaries, judgment, presence, permission, letting go, and enoughness, printing them onto patterned paper, and gluing them down. Coloring intricate mandalas, stapling on ribbon, and adding words about forgiveness. Over my projects, I'd usually felt content, serene, relaxed. Fingers hovering over paint in bubblegum pink, lemon yellow, and calypso teal settled churning thoughts. I was fully present to the moment. And sometimes Faith and I had made art together.

Every so often, I'd flipped back through my journal pages, pleased by bright colors, inspirational words, and playful characters. *Look at me go!* It had been a long time since I'd turned blank paper into something else.

And, because life is rarely a straight line, every so often, I'd critiqued the simplistic art, eviscerating pages I hated. *Stupid. Ugly. You should quit. Why do you bother?*

There were pages I'd thought about ripping to shreds. Abject failures that had caused me to chuck a paintbrush or the glue stick onto the floor. I wanted pretty. I wanted perfect. I wanted to make what the artists on YouTube were making. Well drawn. Well executed. A certain aesthetic. Or, at least, better. More than once, I'd cried out in frustration. More than once, I'd stormed away. *Hack!* I didn't know why I bothered. But each day, I'd shown back up to my art table, excited by the limitless promise of blank paper and colorful supplies.

One month had ticked by. Two, three, four, six. Each time I'd turned to a fresh white page, dozens of times, I'd reminded myself, proved to myself, that I deserved to take up space. To let down my guard. To make my mark. To make art. *I'm worth it.* Once in a while, I'd believed me. The outcome had mattered less than engagement with the process—a process that didn't feel wasteful or boring or stupid. In fact, at my art table, I'd felt energized. Renewed. Restored.

Inside me, abandoned and ignored parts began to peek out from behind the protective barrier of my armor, risking exposure in the hope of receiving respect, acceptance, and love. What those parts might be labeled, "younger versions" or "shadow aspects," matters less than knowing they existed, craved acknowledgment, and desired expression.

I'd only ever understood self-care from the point of view of the outside inward: dieting, exercise, movies, books, mani-pedis. But self-care was meant to be a two-way street—outside in and inside out, an embodied lifestyle.

Now, at my art table, surrounded by paper towels, baby wipes, and alcohol inks, I took a step back. I tilted my head from side to side. A drip hadn't fanned. A drop hadn't trickled. The colors clashed. I could see only the imperfections, the hot mess of it. Not, this time, any of the fun. Red, blue, and green mixed in spots to an unattractive brown, the way those colors can. My throat ached. I scowled. Judgment.

"And if this page turns out to be a failure, so what? What happens?"

I mean, I stood there not for the first time remembering to ask myself these questions out loud.

Failure, I was slowly learning to believe, was only failure because I ascribed that meaning to it. In my art journal, my best efforts were good enough. In my art journal, failure was another word for opportunity. A regular art practice was proving time and again that imperfection often turned out to be my favorite quirk on a page. That tear, those smears, even some muddy brown were an impetus to pivot, to consider a bold new alternative. Or to accept that imperfect is another word for unique, and to leave well enough alone.

Besides, if I called my art, something I made with my head, hands, and heart, with love, "ugly," I might as well look in the mirror and say the same thing to my face. I refused to do that to myself anymore. *Breathe.*

I headed for my stacks of magazines, confident I'd find embellishments for a page that was a work in progress but headed in the right direction.

Like me.

AFTERWORD

NEWBURY PARK, CALIFORNIA
January 2024

Any memoir that highlights a child is a delicate undertaking.

So first, this: I have my family's permission to tell our story. Eleven years have passed since the events depicted in these pages, and the three of us remain committed, in our own ways, to sharing our experiences, demystifying mental health diagnoses, and creating safe spaces for important conversations.

Shortly after Faith's diagnosis, I began writing, mostly in notes and fragments. Back then, as our story was unfolding, I had no intention of going public. In time, I changed my mind. Other families, so many families, were on their own similar journeys. There is community, there can be comfort, in sharing. Enrolling in my first memoir writing class, I began to write in earnest full sentences, dialogue, scenes. I finished that class, worked with one editor and then another. I signed up for more classes, for workshops, and with more teachers. I honed my craft while also broadening the story's scope beyond the facts of one child's illness and her parents' reactions.

Two years, four years, six years. I'd write and I'd stop writing. I kept bumping into limitations. Limitations every writer contends with, like structure, characterization, and aboutness.

And limitations related to the extent, at any given time, of my personal growth.

Sometimes, as if chucking a paintbrush or glue stick, I'd slam my laptop shut, convinced my quest was impossible. I swore. I cried. But for reasons I have trouble articulating still today, our story always called me back to the page, to more classes, and more teachers.

Eight years after Mom's death and Faith's diagnosis, at the start of the COVID-19 pandemic lockdown, I recommitted to a daily writing practice. I was determined to make good use of a terrible time, and to become, finally, someone who finished. Someone who, without a formal writerly education, achieved completion of a book-length project, and who stopped hiding. Most importantly, I wanted to make meaning out of my family's extremely difficult experience. For another year I wrote, and I did find my way to an end. In 2021, I sent that version of the manuscript to my publisher, anticipating a May 2022 release.

But during the days, weeks, and months following that submission, I began to sense in my gut a growing unease. I feared. For myself. For my family. I feared that in spite of my dedicated and prolonged efforts, that version of the story still had not done justice to us or my intentions. I tried to rationalize my fear, telling myself that any first-time memoirist would have nerves. I was reluctant to interrupt the publishing process, concerned that I might never find the necessary bravery and fortitude to recommit, again. Toward the end of 2021, my apprehension reached fever pitch.

With the final deadline for a decision mere days away, I reached out for support. To whom and from where doesn't matter. But I asked people who both did and did not know me, who both knew and knew nothing about the lengths I'd gone to to write our story true, for words of advice and encouragement. I heard from folks I had considered friends, who said terrible and untrue things about my family and me, utterly unconcerned about the veracity of their statements. Assumptions. Fallacies. Inaccuracies. I was threatened with legal action.

Knowing that those words said more about the people saying them than they did us did little to assuage the pain in my heart.

To another specific subset, people who had already done what I was about to do, writers who were bound by their commitment to memoir—I again reached out for help. I was not seeking nor did I expect tacit support or approval. What I wanted was thoughtful, nuanced perspectives. Real-world perspicacity. Insight.

Just two or three people answered the questions I'd asked respectfully. Plenty more, and I mean plenty of others, answered me with judgment. *A mother has no right to say such things, no right to tell such stories. A mother shouldn't treat her child that way, shouldn't ambush her family for monetary gain.*

Money? As if . . .

I was unprepared for the vehemence. My childhood had, as I've made clear, left me particularly vulnerable to rejection. Shame grows in silence. Silence can kill. I was being told, it seemed to me, to chuck my book into a fire.

The attempts to make me small and afraid filled me with doubt. And they worked.

Grief-stricken, I contacted my publisher, pulling the book from release.

Thank goodness.

Thank goodness not because I acquiesced to other people's opinions about what was right for me and my family, but thank goodness because I had been right. I'd listened to my intuition. The distress I'd been feeling was trying to tell me something. My story needed more work.

And so, in 2022, I began again to write. And again, I stopped, wondering if I'd ever be able to honor what my family had been through, and more importantly, where we've ended up. Plus, a memoir's main character is supposed, at least mostly, to be a version of the author's self, but as I wrote and rewrote, I realized the person most missing in the earlier drafts was me.

Another outcome of a childhood like mine is that as an adult I had no idea, almost all of the time, what I was feeling beyond the big, easy-to-identify emotions like anger, fear, or sadness. If an inability to discern emotions seems incongruent with what you've read within these pages, phew! It took a lot of work, therapy, art, and healing, and all the years of writing and rewriting these pages for me to finally understand subtleties related to my past's impact on us around the time of Faith's diagnoses and beyond.

What I mean to say is, year after year, by working at writing, I was working at making my life.

In early 2023, again, I began to write. Finally, I found my way to the end of this book.

I don't have neuroscience research handy to back up my claim, but I believe I had to literally write new brain pathways into existence, write in order to heal conduits, write in order to build a more well-rounded, in-depth, refined version of myself and the story. I wouldn't be who I am without that process of wrestling with words and blank white paper.

There will be as many opinions about the story I've told as those whose fingers touch these pages. I doubt any will be worse than what I, myself, have already thought. *I'm inflicting harm on my daughter. I've sensationalized my daughter's illness. I might be encouraging people "out there" who don't know her to do harm.*

But with my family's support, I have become a woman and writer committed to dispelling judgment—mine and other people's. I am working, every day, to release habituated judgmental thought patterns. I'm committed to normalizing struggles like ours. Mental illness doesn't discriminate. Healthy, appropriate, hope-filled dialogue will always far outweigh the naysayers. Every story shared is proof that we are not alone—or do not have to be.

And as to my bloodlines.

I have much left to unpack and heal around my childhood trauma—my mother's narcissistic neglect and invalidation and my father's codependence and enmeshment, the emotional family system I was born into. These interpersonal dynamics, completely unconscious, compounded by Lauren's death and shrouded in silence and secrecy, set the stage for what I would know and not know about being the type of person and type of parent I longed to be. I am not implying that everything about my childhood was negative. That would be an unfair oversimplification. But, since most if not all of my choices were driven by forces I had no idea existed, I did things I didn't really want to do without understanding why. Like passing out in a bar—one self-harming incident in a long line of escalating incidents that can be traced to trauma.

In an attempt to remove stigma, fear, and shame around mental illness and established constructs of self-harm, I am trying to broaden the view. To say, plainly, that the use of negative coping skills, in whatever form, is commonplace. While there may be a necessary time and place for categorizing behaviors, the truth is we are more alike than we are different. We are people doing our best.

Therapy excavated unhealthy paradigms I recreated with Faith. To be clear, I am not implying that my mothering caused my daughter's mental illness. That would turn back the hands of time to a dangerous point in our history. I am saying that by the time Faith returned home from the second stint in residential treatment, I had had enough experience to conclude that as painful as the truth was, I did not actually possess the power to cure or control her illness. My daughter's healing journey, like her life, was just that—hers.

Within my power to do, the path to being most helpful was by showing up, in the healthiest ways possible, by doing the work to uncover and understand the patterns that had created me, what those forces allowed and didn't allow me to do for others, for myself, and for her. What had trickled down my bloodlines had taught me that safety and love were conditional, vulnerability dangerous. Most of all, my bloodlines had hindered my ability to express and receive love—the pattern I most wanted to rectify.

One small step at a time, I began to recognize unhealthy dynamics—enmeshment, codependence, escapism, people-pleasing, to name a few—and rebuild healthier ones. Not as a mean to the end of curing illness; rather, because healthy relationships, of any kind, form from mutual respect and admiration, not desperate attempts to avoid rejection.

Now, to us.

My husband read these pages, and his assessment of my portrayal of him during the days depicted is, in his words, "accurate." But it would be a mistake to think any of us is still who we were then. Theo's love language is work, being useful and productive. As I type these words, he's outside. Busy painting the exterior of our house, by himself, because that's how he rolls. Doing so, at seventy-three years old, to save money and so I won't have to worry about paint when he's "not around anymore." Our eighteen-year age difference compels him to find ways to take care of me that extend into the future.

Our relationship isn't perfect, of course. No one's is. But we strive to maintain healthier communication, to repair, to remember that words have impact. Theo never stops asking what I need or how he can support me. Every day, we say, "I love you." The pandemic shutdown of the entertainment business forced him into full retirement. We've created a daily routine that suits us both. And he continues to do everything in his power to support Faith.

In the giving back department, for years Theo has been a twelve-step sponsor, using his knowledge and life experience to help others struggling with drug and alcohol addictions. And he volunteers as a high school assistant golf coach, melding a love for the game with a long career as a leader to positively shape teen boys' attitudes about themselves, each other, and life. He's particularly adept at helping kids who are hard on themselves, whose anxious natures impede their ability to enjoy the sport and compete.

As for me. During Faith's high school years, I got involved with our local affiliate of the National Alliance on Mental Illness (NAMI), first as a student and then as a volunteer teacher, presenter, and board member. Through NAMI, I began sharing our story. In churches, schools, and auditoriums. To teachers, parents, and students. I openly shared about life in the aftermath of a child's diagnosis. I've been interviewed by our local newspaper, and I've appeared as a guest on mental health–themed podcasts. At first, I was scared. Would folks judge us, our story, the circumstances, the choices we made? Instead, what I experienced, time and time again, was appreciation. Was gratitude. Relief. Proving to someone young or older that they are not alone had a profound impact on them and on me.

The single most common question people ask me is what one thing—which intervention, technique, person, or place—helped Faith the most. I understand the desire for an easy answer. An obsession with wanting to know what . . . to . . . do. For a long time, I had that same obsession. The problem is, there is no easy answer. And there won't be one any time soon. This journey can last a lifetime.

Punishment isn't and will never be the answer. Nor is ceding to bullies or to the shame that can arise when society persistently closes the door to those fighting invisible challenges. As we deal with the fallout from the COVID-19 pandemic, the metrics of youth mental health are headed in the wrong direction. Google "CDC Youth Risk Behavior Survey 2011–2021." The time for pretending that mental health doesn't exist or for buying into the lie that mental health challenges equate to weakness is over. The time for action is now.

Around the time of Faith's senior year of high school, I started teaching creative art journaling at our local adult school. I still do. While I focus on fun, I try never to miss an opportunity to remind my fellow artists about the beauty of imperfection, the need for self-expression, and the inspiration of art as a balm for the soul. Color theory, design, and aesthetics are the how, not the why. Absolutely, positively, one hundred percent for sure, you do not need to be a "real" artist, whatever that means, in order to create art you enjoy, to be worthy of the benefits of a creative, artistic lifestyle.

I am still overweight and still struggle sometimes to appreciate my body and ignore a lifetime's worth of messaging about looks-based worth. I no longer keep a gratitude list every night, but during low points, I turn to my journal to write about the abundance inside and around me. For years, I've maintained a personal spiritual practice that connects me to myself and others and to making conscious choices that strengthen integrity, love, and compassion.

I'm grateful for the life I have today. I'm most especially grateful for my relationship with my daughter.

Faith graduated from high school with a scholarship to attend one of her top choice universities, where she studied environmental science and theater. Her passion was and remains saving the planet. Upon graduating university, again with honors, she was invited to join Phi Beta Kappa, and was one of two seniors in the environmental science cohort presented with a special award for outstanding performance, participation, and passion in the field.

For two years, Faith lived in San Jose, California, where, as an AmeriCorps fellow with Climate Action Corps, she volunteered, receiving a stipend. She provided in-school education to students, faculty, and staff on environmental conservation. She was the sort of person who went for a walk every day with a big bucket, collecting trash along the way. She was the sort of person who donned a hazmat suit, in the blazing heat, and entered a flood zone to help dig toxic mud out of a family's home. She was and still is the sort of person who has been in a committed relationship (not with the same high school boyfriend) for more than four years.

Not surprisingly, she aims to please, which we discuss on a fairly regular basis. She works hard to be a kind person, a good friend, coworker, and daughter. She doesn't always succeed. No one does. And she continues to heal, learn, and grow, continues to work on understanding her diagnoses and her bloodlines and their impact on her life. In ways big and small, she thrives. Together, we're determined to break trauma's generational chain of transmission. She still knows I've got her back.

Faith supports my desire to share about our experiences so that others will know they are not alone. She read these pages—old enough now, at age twenty-five, to re-experience the difficult times through a more mature, healing lens. Maturity allowed her to commiserate with my sorrow over my complicated relationship with her grandmother, and to appreciate that their relationship was not complicated. Over words on the page we chuckled and sniffled. Faith reminded me that nothing about what happened with her illness was my fault. I reminded her that nothing was her fault either. We talked and we talked some more, and we had, in fact, more meaningful dialogue in the span of a few weeks than I had in a lifetime with my mother. We shared our excitement for and gratitude over our strengthening bond. I am watching her emerge as a young woman with so much future ahead.

We often talk, text, and Zoom. We write letters to one another. We talk about having feelings, what to do when they're painful, how to manage them in healthier ways. I learn from her. We have empathy and compassion for one another, and still sometimes get annoyed. That's life!

Whenever the opportunity presents itself, we spend time together. To Theo and me, Faith says, "I love you." We always say, "I love you" back. I look forward with joy to whatever is yet to come in our mother-daughter relationship. Faith, I know, does too. This connection, to the outside world, may seem common, but for those, like me, who never before experienced it, I can tell you it is downright miraculous.

All my life, I've turned to books for information, insight, inspiration, and promise. Over-analyzing was never going to solve my problems, but books provided invaluable stepping stones on the path to a healthier me. I hope this one provided encouragement for you.

DISCUSSION GUIDE

1. This book is called *Bloodlines*, a word with multiple connotations. How did the title shape your expectations of the story?
2. More people than ever are speaking out about their mental illness. And stigma still exists. What might you do to decrease stigma and increase the likelihood that people who need help reach out for it?
3. Weight and body image are recurring themes in the book. The author is candid about the struggles faced by herself and her daughter. How did the unfolding story change or reinforce your ideas about body image?
4. Is there a behavioral pattern—your own, a loved one's—that you now recognize and understand differently than before? How so?
5. The author suggests that self-care is a two-way street. Do you agree? What would embodied self-care look and feel like to you?
6. The author attempts to cope with her daughter's intensifying behaviors with a variety of coping mechanisms. What are they? Which coping mechanisms do you resort to or rely on when circumstances seem to be spiraling out of control?
7. Reflect on a time when you felt judged. How did you respond? How might you respond differently next time? What do you

wish your family and friends might do differently the next time they feel inclined to judge?

8. What hurdles have you had to overcome in your life so that you might grow more connected to yourself, your family, and friends?

9. For someone who has never received therapy, the prospect can be scary. Has this book changed your perspective on therapy? How so?

10. The author suggests that it is important to make conscious choices about the relationships in your life—to make room for love and to pay attention, even when there seems to be no time. What are some of the ways you work to make room—and what additional opportunities to strengthen your relationships might you pursue?

11. The author shares experiences related to bullying and how difficult it is to take a stand against harmful behavior. What are some consequences related to not speaking up? Have you found ways to use your own voice? When? How? What happened?

12. If you are a parent, did you intend to be a different kind of parent than the one(s) you grew up with? If so, how? What did your childhood teach you about being a parent? Having expectations?

13. Has your view of any failures or shortcomings of your parents or parent figures changed after reading this book? If you were to write of your parents or parent figures, what stories would you tell?

14. Do you believe that trauma carries forward, generation to generation? Have you seen such evidence in your own life?

15. Words are labels, the author suggests. They may fall short, but they also serve a purpose. What labels have you found yourself

relying on to describe an important experience or person? How would your understanding of either shift, were you to use other words?

16. This is the story of a mother who must, in some ways, reinvent her understanding of herself and of her daughter. Which tool(s) do you think she found most useful? Which tools would be most applicable in your life?
17. How did the author's relationship with her daughter change from the beginning of the book to the end? How did she begin to love differently?
18. How would you define compassion? How did the author's understanding of compassion evolve as the story unfolded?
19. If you hit a rough patch with your own mental health, what support would you seek?
20. What questions would you ask the author, were you to meet her in person?

ACKNOWLEDGMENTS

The silliest thought I had when I decided to write this book was, *How hard can it be?* That was thousands of revisions and a boatload of thank-yous ago. To my many writing mentors, I say thank you for the time and effort you put into my writing journey and my life, for rarely tiring of having to give me the same guidance time and again, and for creating safe spaces for women to speak their truth. I'm paying it forward to the best of my ability. I hope I'm honoring you, Laura Munson, Jennie Nash, Beth Bornstein Dunnington, Linda Schreyer, Linda Joy Myers, and Jeannine Ouellette.

Beth Kephart, award-winning author and cofounder of Juncture Writing Workshops, artist, mentor, teacher, facilitator, and friend. Your dedication to the art and craft of writing and living inspired me every day to do better. Without the many versions of you and your generosity, this book in its current form would unequivocally not exist. Thank you for never giving up on me.

Thank you to Brooke Warner and the team at She Writes Press for their dedication to women's stories, and for masterfully shepherding our voices into the world.

Special thanks to the folks at Smith Publicity, Inc., including Corinne Moulder and Joelle Speranza, the team at Marstin, including Abigail O'Richey, and to beta readers extraordinaire: Jeni Driscoll; L. Kris Gowen, PhD; Mary Novaria; and Kimmi Quinn. Thank you. Your generosity lives on every page of this book.

The following people are so special to my family and to me; we wouldn't be who we are without your presence in our lives. Thank you Jade Dearing, Wendy Goldstein, Bob Marks, Terri Palmer, Kimberly Prendergast, Maria Rodgers O'Rourke, Diane Sall, and Shari Schwartz.

To Susan Schwartz, friend, reader, writer, artist, person of big heart and soul, thank you for your love and support, for reading and writing, for seeing in ways that I cannot.

To the mothers who came before me, willing to express what needed expressing, thank you.

To my mother, Lauraine Sullivan, and my father, Gerald Sullivan: You live on in our hearts and minds and are with us every day. I miss you both so much. I love you.

To my husband, whom I can count on no matter what and no matter when, thank you. Thank you for your willingness to be open and honest about our story. I know you believe, as I do, that sharing is a direct route to healing. I love you.

To my daughter: Hundreds of thousands of written words and hundreds of hours of spoken ones barely scratch the surface in expressing what you mean to me. I am who I am because of the gift of you in my life. You are magnificence personified. I love you, to the moon and back.

If you or someone you know is struggling or in crisis, help is available. Call or text 988 or chat 988lifeline.org to reach the 988 Suicide & Crisis Line.

A list of resources can be found at www.traceyyokascreates.com/writing/mental-health-resources/.

ABOUT THE AUTHOR

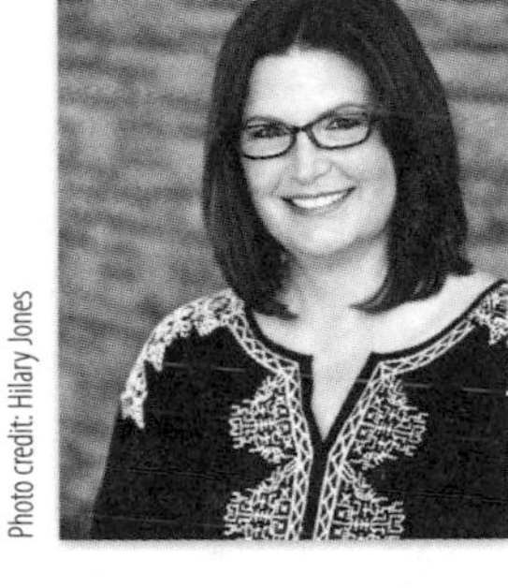
Photo credit: Hilary Jones

Tracey Yokas creates stuff. She is a writer and artist inspired by the intersection of creativity, community, and healing. When she isn't writing about mental health and wellness, she can be found playing with paint, glitter, and glue. She earned her master's degree in counseling psychology from California Lutheran University. Tracey lives in Newbury Park, California, with her family. Visit her website at www.traceyyokascreates.com; she'd love to hear from you. You can also find her on Facebook @traceyyokascreates and Instagram @traceyyokas.

SELECTED TITLES FROM SHE WRITES PRESS

She Writes Press is an independent publishing company founded to serve women writers everywhere. Visit us at www.shewritespress.com.

Canaries Among Us: Parenting at the Intersection of Bullying, Neurodiversity, and Mental Health by Kayla Taylor. $17.95, 978-1-64742-293-6. An urgent exposé revealing the most widespread yet little acknowledged threat to child well-being: lack of acceptance. This daring memoir not only uncovers the truth about how our schools and communities treat unique children but also provides meaningful insights for a more dignified future, through the lens of Taylor's own experiences raising a neurodiverse child.

Emma's Laugh: The Gift of Second Chances by Diana Kupershmit. $16.95, 978-1-64742-112-0. After Diana's first child, Emma, is born with a rare genetic disorder, Diana relinquishes her to an adoptive family, convinced they will parent and love Emma better than she ever could—but when fate intervenes and the adoption is reversed, bringing Emma back home, Diana experiences the healing and redemptive power of love.

Fixing the Fates: An Adoptee's Story of Truth and Lies by Diane Dewey. Since being surrendered in a German orphanage forty-seven years ago, Diane Dewey has lived with her adoptive parents near Philadelphia—loved, but deprived of information about her roots. When her Swiss biological father locates her, their reunion becomes an obsession—and ultimately leads her to the answers, and peace, she's been seeking.

Remember Me As Loving You: A Daughter's Memoir by Kimberly Childs. $16.95, 978-1-63152-157-7. In her search for love and home, Kimberly Childs must find her way through her glamorous, alcoholic mother's world of London and Broadway glitz and her grandparents' Kentucky farm with an outhouse before landing in 1960s San Francisco, where she discovers the serenity of meditation—and her life's path.

Swimming for My Life by Kim Fairley. $17.95, 978-1-64742-255-4. Interweaving a tumultuous family tale of eccentric parents and five kids left to fend for themselves with an eye-opening view of the often-hidden dark side of competitive swimming, this compelling memoir provides a glimpse into the backbreaking and sometimes soul-crushing work necessary to achieve elite status in the competitive swimming world.